About the Author

I0121063

Scott E. Hallgren DO FACP attended medical school at the College of Osteopathic Medicine and Surgery and completed his post graduate medical training in the US Army Medical Corp. He is Board Certified in Internal Medicine and Gastroenterology by the American Board of Internal Medicine and is a Fellow of the American College of Physicians. While in the military he was the Assistant Chief of Gastroenterology and Chief of Endoscopy at Fitzsimons Army Medical Center. He received numerous physician teaching awards and was awarded the Meritorious Service Medal by the US Army. In 1990 Dr. Hallgren left the military for private practice at the Florida Center for Gastroenterology where he is the Vice President. He served as Chief of Endoscopic Services, Chief of Medicine, and Vice Chief of Staff at local hospitals and has been active in the post graduate teaching programs for physicians. His current interest is Health and Wellness Medicine and how to incorporate lifestyle changes, integrated medicine, exercise, and nutrition into a person's daily living in order to improve their health. Dr. Hallgren incorporates Integrated Gastroenterology into the care of his private practice patients.

Introduction

Definition of Wellness and Integrative Medicine

The Basics of Wellness

Wellness and Preventative Medicine Highlights

Wellness

An Individual person's blend of medical, physical, psychological, and spiritual well being

This includes:

- Medical health with control of underlying medical problems
- Physical health with appropriate aerobic conditioning and muscle tone
- Psychological well being with happiness in the work place, with family and friends, and appropriate activities to maintain this well being
- Spiritual well being is the belief in yourself and others. It is your search for the meaning of life. This may be based in religion, nature, music, or community and is different for everyone

Wellness and Integrative Medicine

Medical care which blends multiple modalities to maintain the wellness/health of an individual. All modalities are scientifically validated and/or scientifically reasonable

This includes any combination of:

- Standard Western medicine: Forms the base of medical care for an individual
- Alternative medicine including Eastern/Chinese herbal medicine, Acupuncture, Herbal therapy, and Super Nutritional therapy
- Nutrition/ Diet
- Weight control
- Exercise
- Psychological treatment including stress management
- Smoking and excessive alcohol cessation
- Preventative medicine

Basics of Wellness

The Rocky Mountain Health and Wellness Center guide to wellness and integrative medicine is divided into sections which progressively build information. The initial summary outlines the essence of wellness and a healthy life style, and for the quick reader provides the basic overall thought process. Part I reviews the "nuts and bolts" of wellness and integrated medicine. Reading and understanding these initial suggestions will start you on your journey to wellness. The subsequent sections (Parts II, III, and IV) provide in depth information on a range of wellness and integrative medicine topics and offer information that your primary physician may not suggest. This information combines scientifically proven evidence based western medicine with scientifically proven or reasonable complementary and alternative medicine (CAM). There are many situations where varying combinations of western medicine and eastern/complementary medicine are the best solution to health and wellness. Enjoy the reading as the information will help you develop a happy and healthy lifestyle.

Basics of Wellness

- **Be happy:** Wellness starts with a mentally stable and happy frame of mind. Learn to enjoy the positives that are already in your life and engage in activities that promote enjoyment. Consider the positives of family and friends and find the best part of your day at work, whether in a job or at home, and emphasize this area. Add activities that add enjoyment to your life. This may include religion, watching or participating in athletic activities, art, music, cooking, reading, watching movies, etc. There are many options which promote emotional stability. During times of stress use activities such as meditation, muscle relaxation, relaxed breathing, biofeedback, etc. that are all very helpful in decreasing the stress level. Many activities such as yoga, Tai Chi, and exercise are also stress reducers. The key is to find what works for you and implement these changes. If depression does set in then medical treatment can be extremely beneficial. This may include counseling, super nutritional or herbal therapy, and potentially medical pharmacological therapy.

- **Eat well:** Nutrition is the second building block in overall health and wellness. Start with a healthy eating pattern of 5-6 small "meals" per day with the appropriate intake of lean protein, healthy carbohydrates, and unsaturated fats. Minimize saturated fat and enriched carbohydrates while eliminating Trans fat and Esterified fats. Portions should be controlled although specifically counting calories is not necessary. Learn to cook in a healthy and nutritious fashion at home and when eating out be cautious on the portion size and nutritional make up. Be particularly careful with processed food, fast foods, and overall salt intake. Alcohol and soda add unnecessary additional calories and should be minimized. Understanding the nutritional composition of food makes these decisions much easier.
- **Exercise:** This is another extremely important facet of health and wellness. Regular exercise promotes the release of endorphins which help mental wellness, improves aerobic capacity which allow a feeling of well being along with improving organ health (heart, lungs, etc), and increases muscle tone which also maintains health and simply makes you look better and thereby feel healthier. Exercise includes aerobic activities such as running, fast walking, stationary or street bicycling, treadmill, elliptical, swimming, etc. and anaerobic activities such as weight lifting. It is important to exercise regularly but also vary the sessions in order to maximize the effect and prevent boredom. Athletic activities can substitute for an exercise session and can add enjoyment in your life.
- **Take supplements:** Despite the best nutritional intentions, our diet is still commonly deficient in many areas and supplements can improve overall health. A multiple vitamin with minerals daily provides a big step in insuring appropriate vitamin and mineral intake. Omega 3 supplementation with at least 600 mg of EPA and DHA is heart healthy in addition to multiple other benefits. Since B vitamins can be difficult to find in our diet in recommended doses, a Super B complex is an excellent addition to the multivitamin. Other daily supplements which are reasonable include enteric coated low dose (81mg) aspirin for men over 40 and women over 50, Fiber, and a Probiotic. Considerations can be given to Calcium with Vitamin D (in specific situations), Zinc, Glutamine, Coenzyme Q10, and Vitamin C. Each person needs to individualize their particular needs.
- **Be healthy:** Integrative medicine blends classical western medicine with medically reasonable alternative medicine. It is very important to

establish a trusting relationship with a primary care physician (PCP). The best primary physicians for adults are Internal Medicine Specialists and Family Practice Physicians as these doctors receive superb training in all facets of adult medical care. Research your physician choice carefully by listening to family, friends, and health care ancillary personnel and resist allowing your insurance company to assign your physician. Make sure your choice is board certified in their area of expertise as this is an additional suggestion that the physician is highly qualified. The optimum primary care doctor will be intelligent, up to date, compassionate, and willing to spend the necessary time with your particular health care needs. Discuss their feelings on Integrative medicine as many physicians are reluctant to consider alternative care. The PCP should also be willing to refer to a specialist when medically indicated. Many insurance companies will restrict your choice of a primary care physician as they will have an "approved list." If your initial PCP choice does not meet your needs, change doctors. If you are unable to find the correct physician within their network you may need to change insurance companies. Choose your health care plan with equal caution as today's insurance plans are difficult to comprehend and may be missing important coverage that can affect the quality of your care. Try to blend your needs from a health standpoint with your financial situation. Pay particular attention to the deductable, copay, and out of network expenses as these are "hidden" costs which can add up quickly. Never choose a "capitated" plan which essentially pits your well being in direct conflict with the physician's financial well being. Do not put off having preventative testing done and never ignore a new symptom or a "red flag" symptom which might suggest the onset of a serious disease. Early treatment provides the best chance of reversing the process and re-establishing your health.

- **Change your bad habits:** Smoking, alcohol, and illicit drugs cessation are the three major lifestyle changes which can quickly improve your overall health. The dangers of smoking have been well documented scientifically and include an increased risk of heart attacks and strokes, advanced lung disease with COPD (Chronic Obstructive Pulmonary Disease), peripheral vascular disease, and higher risks of many different cancers including lung, pancreas, esophageal, breast, colon, and bladder. Second hand smoke inhalation has similar devastating effects and should be avoided as much as possible. Discontinuing smoking may reverse the deleterious effects of smoking. If your life partner also smokes it is crucial that both people stop smoking together as this will provide the optimum chance for success. Alcohol is a "two edged sword" with potentially beneficial effects in low amounts and particularly dangerous effects at higher intake levels. The intake of 1-2 small glasses of wine on a several time per week basis appears to have protective effects for the heart. Higher intake levels on a daily basis clearly have major liver effects with the potential for end stage alcoholic liver disease. Moderation is the key. If you already have a drinking problem then abstinence is the only effective treatment. The liver is an organ which can regenerate itself if the damage is not already end stage, therefore early on in life it is extremely important to control your alcohol intake. Illicit drugs overall do not have any useful health benefits and are highly addictive. They should be avoided at all costs. Marijuana may have a health benefit due to its anti-nausea properties, but if used should be medical grade and monitored by a physician.

- **Family genetics:** Many common diseases such as high cholesterol, high blood pressure, heart disease, and diabetes have a degree of genetic predisposition. This inherited component cannot be avoided, but you have the ability to modulate the damage with lifestyle changes. Wellness medicine techniques help delay the onset of chronic medical problems and assist in controlling the severity of the illness once it develops.

Quick tip

These quick tip boxes will be scattered throughout the book and provide short, important suggestions related to the topic. Look for them and enjoy the recommendations.

Wellness and Preventative Medicine Highlights

Eat right and diet right

Healthy eating habits are the key to wellness. Try to achieve and maintain your optimum weight by intelligent changes in your dietary intake that promote wellness. High fat diets (such as the Adkins diet) are rarely the long term answer!!! Children need to learn to eat nutritiously so plan healthy meals and start them on the road to long term wellness.

Fitness

The second key to wellness is fitness. A regular exercise program is vital to your health. Don't forget to include the family in your fitness plan as children also need regular exercise. Instill a love of exercise early in their life and this will lead to a life of wellness. 25% of US children are currently overweight or obese and this obesity trend needs to be reversed!!! Family activities that are fun and promote fitness are crucial.

Stress management

Stress may build up from problems that develop from work, family, financial, relationships, illness, and many other sources. Learn to control stress with meditation, relaxed breathing, or whatever maneuver works for you. Find your stress reliever and use it!!! Plan weekly activities to make you and your family happy and assist in relieving stress. When your relationship is stressed, take a step back and relax. Use Sunday evening to set up your week's schedule (including meals and snacks) in order to minimize your constant daily stress.

Sleep well

Try to insure a good night's sleep on a regular basis as this provides your body with a chance to recharge its engines. Generally 7-9 hours of sleep per night is recommended but you can make up some of this time with naps during the day. When necessary carve out 20 minutes, sit back, and relax. Allow your mind to wander to help relieve stress.

Quit smoking and control excessive alcohol intake

Smoking is clearly a major health threat and second hand smoke from other people is equally dangerous. Many cancer risks skyrocket with smoke exposure and most lung cancer is a direct result of smoking or second hand smoke exposure. Quit so you do not expose your spouse and children to this second hand smoke!!! If you and your spouse both smoke, then it must be a joint effort to quit as it is unlikely one of two smokers attempting to quit will have long term success. Choose a method of quitting, set a date, and get started. Excessive alcohol intake can be equally dangerous from a medical standpoint. If you are drinking daily then you are probably drinking too much.

Oral health care

Regular dental care is important to good health as tooth decay and gum disease can increase your infection risk due to the bacterial content in the mouth. This higher infection rate also increases the overall inflammatory response in the body and increases the incidence of heart disease, stroke, and potentially cancer. Daily brushing and flossing is mandatory with a professional dental cleaning and examination at least yearly. Don't forget to brush your tongue. Oral cancer can be detected earlier with regular examinations with a higher incidence found in men. Tobacco users (particular chewing tobacco) also have a much higher incidence of oral cancer and should be examined twice a year. Better yet, quit smoking or chewing!!!

Strong bones

Women in particular are susceptible to bone loss and this problem accelerates after menopause. It is important to eat foods that are rich in calcium such as milk, yogurt, and broccoli, and consider taking a calcium supplement. Vitamin D is very important in calcium absorption and metabolism so take a calcium supplement that contains vitamin D. People in northern states with less sun exposure are more prone to Vitamin D deficiencies. Higher risk people should have bone density studies.

Flu protection

The flu vaccine is given yearly to protect against the viral strains that are the most likely culprits for that given year. High risk people with significant medical problems and elderly people should clearly have the vaccine yearly. More and more experts are suggesting that all people should have the vaccine yearly. It is safe overall and the flu effects can be devastating. I personally agree that all adults should have the flu vaccine every year.

Skin cancer detection and protection

Most skin cancer is a direct result of sun exposure. Protection is the key with appropriate clothing and/or sun screen. Use a sun screen that protects against both UVA and UVB rays as both may cause a sunburn. The typical sun screen only protects against UVB. Be sure to use at least SPF 15 and cover all exposed area. Don't forget that sunburns can occur on cloudy days so use sunscreen daily. Regular protection will also help slow the sun effects on aging such as premature wrinkling. Watching your skin for suspicious lesions or change in the appearance of a mole is extremely important. Keep an eye on your own skin and help your spouse or partner. Teach your children to use sun screen protection.

Eye care

Glaucoma is excessive pressure in you eyes and can result in sudden blindness. Commonly there are no warning signs so screening by an ophthalmologist or optometrist is the only method for early detection. Make sure your eye pressures are checked at least once between the ages of 40 and 50. If an elevated pressure is detected medical treatment may prevent blindness. Borderline pressures should be followed closely.

Breast health

Mammograms every 1-2 years after the age of 40 and every year after 50 are important in detecting breast cancer early. Self breast exams on a monthly basis are "free" and may help pick up changes in the breast which require earlier evaluation. You can decrease your risk of developing breast cancer by eating healthy, exercising, and stopping smoking. Men, remember you can also develop breast cancer so do not ignore unusual changes in your breasts.

GYN exams

Regular GYN examinations with pap smear should be done within 3 years of becoming sexually active and then every 3 years (some recommendations suggest yearly) until age 65. Cervical cancer is a potentially preventable problem with careful screening. Pap smears are necessary even if you have received the HPV vaccine as you are still at risk for certain types of cervical cancer.

HPV vaccination

Vaccination against HPV is a new option available to young women. HPV is a sexually transmitted virus which can cause cervical cancer. Vaccination against this virus before initial infection can prevent HPV infections and therefore decrease the potential for the development of cervical cancer. The key is early vaccination with the optimum being before the onset of sexual activity. Discuss the vaccine with your daughter when you are talking about safe sex practices.

Colon cancer prevention

Adenomatous colon polyps have the potential over the years to grow and degenerate into colon cancer. Removing these polyps clearly decreases the incidence of colon cancer. Unfortunately these polyps do not cause symptoms and screening is the only method of detection. The most accurate screening technique is colonoscopy which visualizes the colon with an instrument inserted into the rectum. This also allows the removal of the polyps at the time of the procedure. CT Colonography (Virtual colonoscopy) uses a CT scanner to detect colon polyps. People with polyps on CT Colonography then require a regular colonoscopy for polyp removal. Everyone should have a screening colonoscopy at age 50 and then every 5-10 years after this if the exam is negative. The recommendations are different if you have a family history of colon cancer so consult your physician.

Male health

Testicular cancer is very treatable and all men post puberty should do monthly self testicular examinations. Consult your physician for any unusual lesions. For prostate cancer the blood PSA level is an excellent screen. Consider a PSA blood test starting at age 50 and then every 3 years.

Silent diseases

Hypertension (high blood pressure), Hypercholesterolemia (high cholesterol), and Diabetes (high sugar/glucose level) are all treatable medical problems which commonly have minimal or no clinical symptoms. Control of these medical problems will decrease the incidence of heart attacks, strokes, kidney disease, and eye disease. Screening with blood pressure readings, serum (blood) cholesterol levels, and serum (blood) glucose levels should be done at least once in your 20's and then more frequently as the year's pass.

Part I

Wellness Survival Guide

The Quick review

The Basics of Diet and Exercise

The foundation of wellness starts with nutrition and exercise which are both equally important. How we eat and what we eat will determine how our bodies can react to the stresses of life, both medical and emotional. A healthy diet will provide the building blocks to maintain normal body functioning. Exercise promotes optimal functioning of the internal organs of our body including the heart, lungs, and brain along with fine tuning the muscular system to permit optimal musculoskeletal balance. Nutrition and exercise are completely the individual person's responsibility as family genetics do not play a role. The following suggestions are the "tip of the iceberg" but form the main foundation.

Nutrition/Diet

- **Eating patterns**: 4-6 small meals per day including breakfast, midmorning snack, lunch, mid afternoon snack, dinner, and 9PM snack. All meals should be small portions as you do not want to overeat at any time. This pattern will prevent rapid increases in insulin levels which allow sugars to be moved into cells and then converted into fat.
- **Carbohydrates**: Not necessarily low carbs but the correct carbs. The optimum carbohydrates include whole wheat products, fruits, and vegetables. Whole wheat products should replace white bread and white pastas. Fruit and wheat carbs should be concentrated in the first part of the day with the dark green vegetables later in the day.
- **Protein**: Lean proteins are important. These include beef cuts without excessive fat (Sirloin), Lean Hamburger or Maverick Beef, Chicken, Pork Loin, Turkey, Turkey Bacon, Fish, Scallops, Shrimp, Dairy products, and Legumes. Careful with shrimp if your cholesterol is a problem. Evening snacks with Casein protein which is a long acting protein are excellent. Examples include low fat mozzarella sticks and low fat cottage cheese.
- **Fat**: Should be limited but not eliminated. Small portions of fat will ensure adequate satiety (full feeling) and prevent overeating of empty calories. Monounsaturated fats with Olive or Canola oil or polyunsaturated fats are the preferred choices. Saturated fats should be obtained from dietary

sources such as dairy, meat, fish, and eggs and the amount should be monitored. Always avoid Trans fats and Esterified fats as they do not have any health benefit.

- **Processed food**: It is important to be careful processed foods as they may have hidden sugar components, commonly have added saturated and trans fats, and they are also very high in sodium. This is a common problem in "fast foods." Careful with "nutritional bars" such as granola, etc as they may add high fructose corn syrup. Special K Bars are an excellent simple choice for a breakfast/nutritional bar.

Quick tip

Remember: Correct Carbs!!! Low fat protein source!!! Unsaturated fats in controlled amounts!!! These are the basics of wellness nutrition and weight management.

- **Alcohol and Regular Soda**: Essentially empty calories. Try to avoid as much as possible.
- **Fluid**: Plenty of water and other fluids are extremely important.
- **Caffeine**: Careful with excess caffeine intake as this will speed up your metabolism. A "faster" metabolism may promote weight loss but will also provide additional stress to your heart and other organs and may elevate your blood pressure. The best option is to speed up your metabolism in healthy ways such as exercise.
- **Cheat meal**: Once you are at your goal weight and wellness, consider one meal per week where you eat your favorite foods which do not fit into a healthy diet. This should be on a set day each week (such as dinner Friday or Saturday night) and this will allow you to put off excessive eating desires when they occur on others days. The cheat day should not be used if you are attempting to lose weight.
- **Patience**: It is common to feel somewhat sluggish in the initial 2 weeks of changing your diet, even though the change is for the best. After this

your energy level will progressively improve and within 6 weeks you will feel like a new person.

Quick tip

Frequent smaller meals and snacks with the correct food choices form the basis of a healthy diet and overall wellness. Do not obsess too much on the actual calorie count but remember that most people underestimate how many calories are in their diet. Take your best guess of your total daily calories and then add 25% to your count. This will be a more accurate estimate of your true caloric intake.

Exercise:

- **Insure adequate medical clearance first.** This is particularly important in people who have had a sedentary lifestyle for an extended time. Consult your regular physician for their opinion on what medical evaluation is necessary.
- **Aerobic**: Exercise 3-4 times per week with 15-45 minutes per session for wellness, but for optimum weight loss 6 times per week is necessary. Aerobic fitness sessions are additive over the course of the day, i.e. three 15 minute **hard** workout sessions are equivalent to 45 minutes. Options include power walking, running, bicycling, stationary biking (consider semi-recumbent for less strain on the back and joints), treadmill, elliptical machine, Stairmaster, running in a pool, swimming, etc. The best option is running, but of all exercises this causes maximum joint stress. Excellent second choices are the semi-recumbent bike, running in a pool, or the elliptical machine. The goal is to elevate your heart rate for an extended period of time. When your heart rate returns to a normal level quickly after an exercise session, this generally indicates a good fitness level and a lower resting heart rate (50-65 beats/minute) also suggests a higher fitness level.

- **Anaerobic**: Weight lifting 2-3 times per week is important as this provides muscle tone which is crucial in overall fitness. Muscle requires more energy than fat to maintain its structure and therefore inherently burns more calories which is beneficial. Additionally, after the anaerobic phase of weight lifting, your body converts to an aerobic phase for several hours which results in long periods of caloric consumption. Weight lifting does not require an expensive gym as simple dumbbells and a Swiss ball can be used to work out all muscle groups. It is important to lift weights correctly to prevent injury.
- **Combined Aerobic and Anaerobic work outs**: It is best to complete the aerobic portion of the work out first. This will initiate the burning of calories and the anaerobic portion will be more beneficial.
- **Sedentary work place:** Recent data suggests that enzymes quickly shut down when sitting and working. Minimal exercise such as walking to the copy machine will reactivate these enzymes. Consider a short walk before lunch and use the stairs rather than the elevator.
- **Patience:** When starting an exercise program start slow and slowly build up the frequency and intensity of your aerobic and anaerobic exercises. Each week you will notice an improvement in your overall well being. Achieving a high fitness level takes 3-6 months depending on what level you were at initially. The lower the initial fitness level the longer it will take. Once you have achieved your desired level, it is important to exercise regularly to maintain this fitness. Everyone has down periods where work or life stresses make it difficult to exercise and the key during this time is to push your self with exercise sessions 1-2 times per week. This will insure that your wellness/fitness level does not deteriorate during these "down times," and you do not waste the hard work you put in at the outset.

Quick tip

Exercise is equally important to nutrition for overall wellness. It is very important to combine aerobic and anaerobic regiments for the optimum results.

Basic Supplement Review

Nutrition obtained through correct food intake is the key, but despite the best intentions our diets will commonly be deficient in various nutrients. Vitamin supplements are essential, but other nutritional supplements also may help balance our metabolism, improve body function, decrease inflammation, and lower the risks of medical problems. Each person needs to select the supplements that are most beneficial for their lifestyle and medical condition. The next section helps guide you in your selections.

Supplement review:

- **Fiber supplement**: 3-5 grams per day in a powder or chewable tablet form: Improves intestinal function, decreases the formation of colonic diverticulosis, and decreases cholesterol. Should be an adjunct to a high fiber diet as daily fiber intake should be 20-30 grams. Benefiber powder is my personal favorite as it is tasteless, can be added to any food or drink without changing the consistency of the substance.
- **Multiple Vitamins with Minerals**: One per day in a tablet or capsule form. Centrum with minerals is an excellent choice.
- **Omega 3/Fish oil**: 800-1500mg per day in a capsule form with a minimum of 600mg of the EPA and DHA omega 3. The liquid form rarely contains sufficient omega 3 without taking large amounts. This supplement will lower cholesterol and triglycerides, decreases platelet aggregation, has anti-inflammatory properties, and increases HDL. Higher doses of Omega 3 may be used as a medical treatment for lipid problems (particularly high triglycerides) but should be supervised by a physician. Lovaza is an example of a pharmaceutical grade Omega 3.
- **Super B Vitamins/B complex**: One per day in a tablet form. It is difficult to obtain adequate B vitamins in a normal diet, therefore supplementation is crucial. This commonly provides an energy boost.
- **Probiotics** (Acidophilus or equivalent intestinal bacteria): Supplement with 2-30 billion bacteria per day in a tablet or capsule form (the refrigerated liquid form is excellent but does not provide any additional benefits over the tablets and is more expensive). Probiotics improve intestinal function,

decrease gas and bloating, and promotes a healthy intestinal bacterial flora. The best is to find a supplement with acceptable numbers of bacteria so only one tablet is needed per day. My favorites pharmaceutical grade probiotics include Align, Flora Q, Florastar, and Culturelle, but there are many off brands which are equally good and will save you money. Ask your Pharmacist about their recommendations as to the best off brands that they stock but make sure they suggest the correct dosage. Save money and still obtain high quality probiotics by going to GNC, Vitamin Shoppe, or another supplement store such as these.

- **Enteric/ Safety coated Aspirin:** 81mg per day in an enteric/safety coated capsule form. Men greater than 40 years old, women greater than 50, and people with significant cardiac risk factors (hypertension, diabetes, hypercholesterolemia, smoking, family history of cardiac disease) should take one per day. It is important to be sure the aspirin is safety coated in order to decrease the risks of gastrointestinal complications (particularly bleeding ulcers). People with high risks of gastrointestinal bleeding (over 65 years old, prior GI bleeding from aspirin related ulcers, ulcer symptoms after starting the medication) may need to consider taking a proton pump inhibitor (Prilosec OTC or equivalent) to help prevent ulcer formation. If you are taking a nonsteroidal anti-inflammatory drug (Motrin or equivalent) with the aspirin, this may also increase the risk of ulcer formation and a proton pump inhibitor may be beneficial in preventing ulcer formation.

- **Coenzyme Q10:** 100 mg per day in a capsule form. This supplement improves oxygen conversion in muscle cells, decreases fatigue, improves energy, and may help in chronic fatigue. Additional data suggests that this supplement has beneficial heart effects and improves cardiac function.

- **Chromium picolinate:** 400 mcg per day in a capsule form. Will improve insulin sensitivity, help normalize blood sugar, and decreases the urge to consume sugar. Chromium may be beneficial in weight loss and in improving diabetic glucose control.

- **Zinc:** 10-25 mg per day in a capsule form. Zinc help to repair intestinal tissue, has anti-inflammatory and antibacterial properties, and helps in colds and flu. It is most beneficial in treating the common cold and in patients with intestinal problems such as Crohn's disease.

- **Glutamine:** 2-5 grams once or twice per day in a capsule or powder form. A supplement that repairs intestinal tissue and has fat burning properties.

It is helpful in weight loss situations for the fat burning effects and in intestinal problems, particularly infectious diarrhea.

- **Vitamin C**: 500 mg per day in a tablet or capsule form. An excellent antioxidant, may help control infection, helps make collagen in bones, teeth, gums, and blood vessels, promotes nitrous oxide formation (helpful with muscle formation), and helps muscle growth. Older data suggests a beneficial effect in the common cold.

- **Calcium with Vitamin D:** 1500 mg calcium per day with Vitamin D in a capsule or chewable form. The supplement must be taken in divided doses 2-3 times per day.   It is best for peri or post menopausal women, people who live in northern states without significant milk or other fortified food intake, and people taking steroids.

Muscle Stack: Designed for the exercise oriented looking for muscle growth: May use all three in combination post exercise, or may use individually. All three groups promote the building of lean muscle but only if combined with appropriate weight training. Supplements will not build muscle without exercise.

- **Whey protein**: 5 grams (consider combining with Casein protein 5 grams). Very safe with excellent results.

- **Creatine**: 5 grams per day. Creatine is extremely safe with multiple potentially beneficial medical effects. The past and active research on creatine is extensive.

- **Nitrous Oxide stimulation**: Arginine (3-5 grams) with Vitamin C (500 mg). There are many other nitrous oxide stimulants but Arginine is the classic. Safety data is less clear but no obvious problems have been reported.

Fat Burning

- **Conjugated Linoleic Acid (CLA):** 3-4 grams per day for maintenance. CLA is best used after weight and fat loss has been achieved as it helps maintain the fat loss. This supplement does not appear to have any direct fat burning capabilities.

- **Chromium picolinate**: 400 mcg per day. As noted above, has fat burning capability along with assistance in glucose control.
- **Stacking- for fat burning**: Arginine (3-5 grams), Glutamine (5-10 grams), GABA – Gamma aminobutyric acid (2-5 grams). The maximum effect is obtained with a dose after exercise and at bedtime.

Combined Stacking for muscle growth and fat burning: This stacking regiment is taken after exercise and is my personal favorite for the exercise motivated person.

- **Combine post work out**: Arginine 3-5 grams, Whey protein 5 grams, Casein protein 5 grams, Creatine 5 grams, Glutamine 5 grams, and Vitamin C 500 mg.

Quick reference survival guide to Wellness

This section is designed to provide a quick reference guide for overall health and wellness. Specific details can be found in subsequent chapters. The initial portion outlines the recommendations which pertain to all people interested in wellness, and the subsequent sections breakdown recommendations for specific levels and specific medical needs:

- ✓ **Novice level**
- ✓ **Intermediate level**
- ✓ **Advanced level**
- ✓ **Heart healthy**
- ✓ **Cholesterol healthy**
- ✓ **Gastrointestinal healthy**
- ✓ **Bone health**
- ✓ **Infection prevention**
- ✓ **Weight loss**
- ✓ **Muscle gain**

Nutrition and Exercise:

- **Basics of diet and exercise:** Refer to this section for details as nutrition and exercise form the foundation of wellness. 5-6 small meals per day with appropriate carbohydrate, lean protein, and unsaturated fats with a smaller amount of saturated fats. Exercise on a regular basis with aerobic and anaerobic sessions.

Lifestyle modification:

- **Stress management:** Control stress with meditation, relaxed breathing, or whatever maneuvers work the best for you.
- **Sleep well:** Insure a good night's sleep on a regular basis.

Injury prevention:

- **Safety belts:** Lap and shoulder belts should be used in both front and back seats for all passengers in a car and if possible in a bus and other forms of transportation. Front and side air bags are also very important.
- **Helmets:** Head protection at all times for motorcycle, bicycle, and ATV use.
- **Firearms:** Safe storage of firearms to prevent unintended use is crucial particularly if small children are in the house or may visit the house.
- **Smoke and CO (Carbon monoxide) detectors:** Should cover the entire house.
- **Alcohol:** Minimal to no alcohol use when using any type of vehicle, bicycling, or swimming. Make sure you have a designated driver or plan on taking a cab if you are planning on consuming alcohol and need to use a vehicle to get home.
- **Sun exposure:** All exposed skin areas including your lips need appropriate constant protection with sun screen or clothing with SPF 15 to 45 recommended. Bald men remember to protect the top of your head. Cloudy days are equally dangerous for sun exposure and reflection of ultraviolet rays off of snow is also quite significant. Also make sure to protect your cornea (eyes) with polarized sun glasses.

Health screening:

- **History and Physical examination:** Should include height and weight with a BMI (Body Mass Index) calculation. Also should include skin cancer screening, depression screening, and hearing/vision screening. Suggested every 5 years starting at age 25.
- **Blood pressure check:** Every 2 years starting at age 20.
- **Diabetes and Lipid screening:** Glucose and cholesterol/LDL/triglycerides/HDL checks at age 25, 35, 45, and then every 5 years.
- **Women' health:** Self breast examinations monthly with physician examination at each GYN exam. Mammograms every 1-2 years for women over 40 and yearly over 50, pap test every 3 years from onset of sexual activity until age 65, Chlamydia screen for sexually active women

under 25 or high risk women at any age, and one density for women over 65.

- **Men's health:** Self testicular examinations on a monthly basis for men after puberty and physician examination with each regular physical. PSA blood level for prostate cancer starting at 50 to 55.
- **Oral health:** Daily brushing and flossing (or water pic) with a professional dental cleaning and examination yearly. Don't forget to brush your tongue. The exam should include an examination for oral cancer.
- **Eye care:** Eye pressure check for glaucoma at least once between the ages of 40 and 50.
- **Colorectal health:** Colonoscopy at age 50 and then every 5 to 10 years if the initial examination is negative. Earlier screening is there is a positive family history of colon cancer in a first degree relative.

Vaccinations:

- **Influenza:** Yearly flu vaccines are strongly suggested for all adults. The vaccine is mandatory over age 65, in people with significant medical problems, or in high risk occupations.
- **Hepatitis A and B:** Suggested for everyone.
- **Tetanus/Diphtheria (Td):** Recommended for everyone with the initial 3 dose series and then a booster every 10 years.
- **Pneumococcal:** Recommended at age 65, for people with significant medical problems, and people who have had a splenectomy. The vaccine should be repeated every 5 years.
- **Shingles:** Recommended at age 60 even if you had Shingles (Herpes Zoster) in the past.

Sexual behavior:

- **Contraception and STD education/screening:** Important in overall health. Prevent unintended pregnancy with appropriate contraceptives and use condoms when you are not in a long term monogamous relationship.

Health risk modification:

- **Smoking cessation:** The single most important risk modification which will help promote wellness.
    - ✓ Decide to stop smoking and set a date.
    - ✓ Control your stress level.
    - ✓ Will power: Plan one day at a time.
    - ✓ Enlist family and friends to help.
    - ✓ Keep your hands and mouth busy.
    - ✓ Brush your teeth after meals.
    - ✓ Avoid alcohol and bars as this will decrease will power.
    - ✓ Promise yourself a reward for success.
    - ✓ Get your significant other to quit smoking with you.
    - ✓ Consider pharmacological help- herbal or prescription.
- **Alcohol cessation:** Another very important risk modification particularly if there is excessive intake.
    - ✓ Admit you have a problem.
    - ✓ Decide to stop drinking and set a date.
    - ✓ Will power: Plan one day at a time.
    - ✓ Enlist family and friends to help.
    - ✓ Change your social activities to decrease the peer pressure to drink and avoid bars.
    - ✓ Get your significant other to quit drinking with you.
    - ✓ Consider changes your "friends" that continue to push you to drink.
    - ✓ Consult your physician for medical assistance.
    - ✓ Promise yourself a reward for success.
- **Illicit drugs:** Never a good idea from any viewpoint. Cessation recommendations are the same as with alcohol cessation.

Novice level wellness

The novice level provides a superb start to overall wellness. If you never progress beyond this level you life will still improve dramatically and you will feel significantly better. Start with the above listed wellness suggestions and add the following:

- **Exercise:** Combine aerobic and anaerobic (weight lifting) exercise with 3-4 sessions per week each lasting a minimum of 45 minutes. 30 minutes should be devoted to aerobic exercise, and 15 minutes to weight lifting. My recommendation for aerobic exercise is a semi-recumbent bike as this causes the least stress on your joints and back. You can also easily read or watch TV which helps pass the time. Anaerobic exercise involves simple weight lifting with a set of dumbbells and a Swiss ball. You need to determine the weight that suits you and work from there. Slowly increase your weight level as your strength increases. The weight you choose should tire you out at the end of the set.
- **Supplements- taken daily:**
  - ✓ Multiple vitamin with minerals: One per day.
  - ✓ Omega-3: 1500 mg per day with at least 600mg of EPA and DHA.
  - ✓ Enteric (safety) coated aspirin: 81 mg per day for men over 40 years of age, women over 50, and people with cardiac risk factors.

Intermediate level wellness

The intermediate level is an excellent long term goal as this will provide a high level of fitness combined with an excellent supplement schedule. This requires some degree of motivation particularly if you have a tough work schedule, but it is worth it. Start with the initial wellness suggestions and add the following:

- **Exercise:** Combine aerobic and anaerobic (weight lifting) exercise with 4-5 sessions per week each aerobic session lasting a minimum of 45 minutes. Aerobic exercise may include combinations of semi-recumbent bike, running, fast walking, elliptical machine, swimming, or any number of outdoor activities. Vary your aerobic exercise routine. I would suggest 30 minutes on a semi-recumbent bike and 15 minutes running or on an elliptical machine. Use the elliptical machine if you have hip, knee, or ankle problems as this will create less stress on these joints with the same work out as running. The sessions can be at different times of the day if this fits your schedule better. Weight lifting should last 30 minutes and use free weights, weight machines, or dumbbells and a Swiss ball. You need to determine the weight that suits you and work from there. Slowly increase the weight level as your strength increases. The weight you choose should tire you out at the end of the set. 8 reps are heavier weights designed to build muscle mass, 10 reps are a slightly lower weight for muscle mass and definition of your muscle, and 15 reps are a lower weight for muscle definition.

- **Supplements- taken daily:**
    - ✓ Multiple vitamin with minerals: One per day.
    - ✓ Omega-3: 1500 mg per day with at least 600mg of EPA and DHA.
    - ✓ Super B complex: One per day.
    - ✓ Enteric (safety) coated aspirin: 81 mg per day for men over 40 years of age and women over 50.
    - ✓ Calcium with Vitamin D: 1500 mg of calcium per day in divided doses for peri or post menopausal women. Also consider this supplement in people who live in northern states with insufficient sun exposure.

Advanced level wellness

The advanced level requires a high level of motivation but will provide fantastic results. Start with the initial wellness suggestions and add the following:

- **Exercise:** Aerobic exercise sessions 5-6 times per week with each each aerobic session lasting 1 hour. Remember you may split the workout into 2 separate sessions per day with 30 minutes per session. My suggestion is the first session should be initially in the AM before work with the second session immediately after work before eating a reasonable dinner. Combine aerobic modes daily such as semi-recumbent bike for 30 minutes and elliptical machine for 30 minutes or change the exercise mode on a weekly basis. Running and the elliptical machine provide the maximum aerobic fitness. Anaerobic (weight lifting) sessions 4 times per week with each lasting 1 hour. Free weights, weight machines, or dumbbells and a Swiss ball. You need to determine the weight that suits you and start from there. Slowly increase the weight level as your strength increases. The weight you choose should tire you out at the end of the set. 8 reps are heavier weights designed to build muscle mass, 10 reps with a slightly lower weight are for muscle mass and muscle definition, 15 reps are a lower weight for muscle definition.

- **Nutrition:** Be sure to add extra carbohydrates post heavy exercise to replace the muscle glycogen burned during the session. This is also a great time to add a protein drink/supplement if you are trying to increase your muscle mass. My suggestion is a protein supplement with both Whey protein (fast acting) and Casein protein (slower absorption).

- **Supplements- taken daily:**
  - ✓ Multiple vitamin with minerals: One per day.
  - ✓ Omega-3: 1500 mg per day.
  - ✓ Super B complex: One per day.
  - ✓ Enteric (safety) coated aspirin: 81 mg per day for men over the age of 40 and for women over 50.
  - ✓ Calcium with Vitamin D: 1500 mg calcium per day in divided doses for peri or post menopausal women. Also consider this supplement in people who live in northern states with insufficient sun exposure.
  - ✓ Fiber supplement: 3-5 grams per day.
  - ✓ Probiotic: 2-30 billion per day.
  - ✓ Coenzyme Q10: 100 mg per day.
  - ✓ Green tea: One cup per day. Provides antioxidants and fat burning.

Quick tip

My suggestion is to start with the novice or intermediate level and increase your level of participation as you experience the beneficial effects of the program. Make sure you slowly increase your exercise level in order to prevent injury and be sure that your primary care physician has medically cleared you for participation in an exercise program.

Heart wellness

Start with the initial suggestions and then add the following:

- **Exercise:** Before embarking on an exercise problem, be sure you are cleared by your Cardiologist. Aerobic exercise sessions should be done 5-6 times per week. Slowly increase your level up to 1 hour per session. The base exercise should be a semi-recumbent bike but vary your routine with fast walking, running, elliptical machine, swimming, etc. Anaerobic (weight lifting) should be done 3-4 times per week with 30 minutes per session. This can be simple with dumbbells and a Swiss ball or more advanced with free weights or machines. You need to determine the weight that suits you and start from there. Slowly increase the weight as your strength increases. The weight you choose should tire you out at the end of the set.
- **Nutrition:** Be particular attentive to a low fat diet (primarily unsaturated fats with a small amount of saturated), high fiber (whole wheat, fruits, and vegetables), and low salt (4 grams per day which is a no added salt diet).
- **Supplements- taken daily:**
    - ✓ Multiple vitamin with minerals: One per day.
    - ✓ Omega-3: 1500 mg per day with at least 600mg of EPA and DHA.
    - ✓ Coenzyme Q10: 100 mg per day.
    - ✓ Super B complex: One per day
    - ✓ Enteric (safety) coated aspirin: 81 mg per day.
    - ✓ Fiber supplement: 3-5 grams per day.

Cholesterol wellness

Start with the initial suggestions and then add the following:

- **Exercise:** Same as the heart healthy suggestions.
- **Nutrition:** Same as the heart healthy suggestions.
- **Supplement- taken daily:**
    - ✓ Multiple vitamin with minerals: One per day.
    - ✓ Omega-3: 1500-3000 mg per day with at least 600mg of EPA and DHA.
    - ✓ Coenzyme Q10: 100 mg per day.
    - ✓ Red yeast rice: 1.2-2.4 grams per day in divided doses.
    - ✓ Super B complex: One per day.
    - ✓ Enteric (safety) coated aspirin: 81 mg per day.
    - ✓ Fiber supplement: 3-5 grams per day.

Quick tip

If you have the potential for heart problems and you are embarking on a wellness program, it is crucial to obtain appropriate medical clearance from your primary care physician or a cardiologist. This clearance is particularly important for the exercise component of your program. A cardiac stress test may be necessary.

Gastrointestinal wellness

Start with the initial suggestions and add the following:

- **Exercise:** Choose novice, intermediate, or advanced wellness recommendations.
- **Nutrition:** Emphasis to a high fiber diet (whole wheat, fruits, and vegetables).
- **Supplements- taken daily:**
    - ✓ Multiple vitamin with minerals: One per day.
    - ✓ Omega-3: 1500 mg per day with at least 600mg of EPA and DHA.
    - ✓ Super B complex: One per day.

- ✓ Probiotics: 2-30 billion per day.
- ✓ Fiber supplement: 3-5 grams per day.
- ✓ Glutamine: 2-5 grams per day.
- ✓ Zinc: 10-25 mg per day.
- ✓ Enteric (safety) coated aspirin: 81 mg per day in men over the age of 40 and women over 50.

Bone wellness

Start with the initial suggestions and add the following:

- **Exercise:** Aerobic sessions 5-6 times per week lasting a minimum of 30 minutes with anaerobic (weight lifting) sessions 3-4 times per week with 30 minutes per session.
- **Nutrition:** Add extra daily products if tolerated. If lactose intolerance is a problem take 2 Lactaid tablets before meals.
- **Supplements- taken daily:**
  - ✓ Multiple vitamin with minerals: One per day
  - ✓ Omega-3: 1500 mg per day with at least 600mg of EPA and DHA.
  - ✓ Super B complex: One per day.
  - ✓ Enteric (safety) coated aspirin: 81 mg per day for men over the age of 40 and women over 50.
  - ✓ Calcium with Vitamin D: 1500 mg of calcium per day in divided doses. Have your physician check your Vitamin D level as extra supplementation may be necessary.

Infection prevention and wellness

Start with the initial suggestions and then add:

- **Exercise:** Choose novice, intermediate, or advanced level wellness recommendations.
- **Nutrition:** Emphasize fruit and vegetable intake in your diet.
- **Supplementation- taken daily:**
    - ✓ Multiple vitamin with minerals: One per day.
    - ✓ Omega-3: 1500 mg per day with at least 600mg of EPA and DHA.
    - ✓ Super B complex: One per day.
    - ✓ Vitamin C: 500 mg to 2 grams per day. Consider dividing the doses to twice a day.
    - ✓ Zinc: 10-25 mg per day.
    - ✓ Green tea: One cup per day.
    - ✓ Enteric (safety) coated aspirin: 81 mg per day in men over the age of 40 and women over 50.

Weight loss and wellness

Start with the initial suggestions and add the following:

- **Exercise:** Aerobic exercise 6 times per week with one hour per session. Remember it is acceptable to split the workout into 2 different sessions per day with 30 minutes hard work out per session. My suggestion would be a session initially in the morning before work, and a second session immediately after work before eating a small, reasonable dinner. Anaerobic (weight lifting) 4-5 times per week with 30 minutes per session. You need to determine the weight that suits you and start from there. Slowly increase the weight as your strength increases. The weight you choose should tire you out at the end of the set. Remember that muscle weighs more than fat and as you tone up your muscle mass will increase. Initially you may not lose the pounds as fast due to the muscle mass, but you will look and feel better. Rather than fixating on you exact weight, look at how you clothes are fitting and how you look in the mirror.

- **Nutrition:** Extra emphasis to watching your caloric intake carefully. Make sure you have 5-6 small meals per day with an emphasis to fruit, vegetables, whole wheat products, lean meat, and unsaturated fat. Breakfast and snacks are extremely important to insure there are no excessive spikes in your insulin levels.
- **Supplements- taken daily:**
  - ✓ Multiple vitamin with minerals: One per day.
  - ✓ Omega-3: 1500 mg per day.
  - ✓ Super B complex: One per day.
  - ✓ Fiber supplement: 3-5 grams per day.
  - ✓ Chromium picolinate: 400 mcg per day.
  - ✓ Glutamine 2-5 grams with Vitamin C 500 mg after each workout.
  - ✓ CLA (Conjugated Linoleic Acid): 3-4 grams per day after the weight loss has been achieved. This will help maintain the fat loss.
  - ✓ Enteric (safety) coated aspirin: 81 mg per day in men over the age of 40 and women over 50.
  - ✓ Optional fat burning stack: Arginine 3-5 grams, Glutamine 5 grams, and GABA (Gamma aminobutyric acid) 2-5 grams after exercise sessions and in the evening before sleep.

Muscle gain and wellness

Start with the initial suggestions and then add the following:

- **Exercise:** Aerobic exercise 6 times per week with 1 hour per session. Remember you may split the workout into 2 sessions on the same day. The first session should be initially in the AM before work with the second session immediately after work before eating a reasonable dinner. Anaerobic (weight lifting) should be a major emphasis with 6 sessions per week. The length of each session should be at least 1 hour but depending on your goals may last up to 3-4 hours. Different muscle sets should be worked at different times in order to promote maximum muscle growth.

- **Nutrition:** Extra emphasis should be given to high quality protein intake. Be sure to take in sufficient carbohydrates before and after the exercise sessions to insure adequate muscle glycogen replacement.
- **Supplements- taken daily:**
  - ✓ Multiple vitamin with minerals: One per day.
  - ✓ Omega-3: 1500 mg per day.
  - ✓ Super B complex: One per day.
  - ✓ Chromium picolinate: 400 mcg per day.
  - ✓ Easy stack: Arginine 3-5 grams, Whey protein 5 grams, Casein protein 5 grams, Creatine 5 grams, Glutamine 5 grams, and Vitamin C 500mg after each weight lifting session and in the evening before sleep.
  - ✓ Enteric (safety) coated aspirin: 81 mg per day in men over the age of 40 and women over 50.

Quick tip

Wellness needs to be an individual long term endeavor. Pick the level of interest you will maintain initially and then work hard to optimize the recommendations within this level. Once you realize how much better you feel, increase the level of participation. Have fun on your road to health and wellness!!!

Protein, Carbohydrate, and Fat Information

Daily suggestions for protein, carbohydrate, and fat intake

Protein: 10-25% of total daily caloric intake

Carbohydrates: 50-60% of total daily caloric intake

Fat: 15-25% of total daily caloric intake

Protein

Proteins are linear chains of amino acids connected by bonds called peptide bonds. Each type of protein has a unique amino acid (aa) sequence. There are 20 amino acids of which 8 are "essential" and cannot be produced by the body. The essential aa include leucine, isoleucine, valine, threonine, methionine, phenylalanine, tryptophan, and lysine. Proteins are important in muscle formation and function, skin and bone support, immune protection, and nerve transmission. Enzymes and most hormones are proteins. Generally recommended protein doses are 1 gram of protein per kg of body weight per day. Extra protein intake is safe unless underlying renal (kidney) problems exist which prevent adequate clearing of unnecessary protein. Advanced liver disease with extra protein intake may result in encephalopathy (mentation/thought problems).

- **Dietary protein:** High quality protein contains all of the essential amino acids.
    1. **Egg protein:** This source of protein is considered the optimum and least expensive. The American Heart Association has stated that one egg per day is acceptable. The white part of the egg contains the protein and the yolk contains the fat, but the yolk also has many other important and excellent nutrients.
    2. **Meat protein (white chicken, white turkey, pork tenderloin, lean beef, fish, and seafood):** Meat is also considered an excellent protein source with chicken, turkey, and fish particularly good due to the lower fat content.

3. **Dairy protein (milk, yogurt, and cheese):** Dairy products contain casein protein which is a long acting high quality protein.
4. **Soy:** This is a plant protein which is considered equal in quality to meat.
5. **Plant protein:** This protein is considered low quality as different plant sources will be lacking in different essential amino acids (remember essential aa must be obtained from dietary sources). If you are a vegetarian then be careful to combine different plants products in your diet in order to obtain adequate intake of all of the essential amino acids. Plant protein examples include legumes (beans with excellent fiber content) and nuts. One cup of beans has the equivalent protein content to 3 oz of steak.
6. **Protein supplements:** Whey protein powder and Casein protein powder (or a combination) can be added to nutritional supplement drinks and smoothies to improve their nutritional value. These protein supplements are an excellent choice for pre and post work out nutritional support.

Carbohydrates

The three main carbohydrates include starch (or complex carbohydrates), sugar, and fiber. Total carbohydrates listed on a nutrition label are the combination of all three.

- **Starch (complex carbs):** These include the following categories:
    1. Starchy vegetables such as green peas, corn, lima beans, and potatoes.
    2. Dried beans, lentils, and peas such as pinto beans, kidney beans, black eyed peas, and split peas.
    3. Grains such as wheat, oats, barley, and rice. The grain group can be broken into whole grain or refined grains. A grain contains three parts: the bran, germ, and the endosperm. The bran contains fiber, B vitamins, and minerals and is the hard outer layer. The germ is the second layer and contains essential fatty acids and vitamin E. The inner core is the endosperm and contains the starch content of the

grain. Whole grain products contain all three layers and therefore all of the nutrients whereas refined grain products only contain the endosperm layer and therefore only the starch. When reading a nutrition label with whole grain products the first ingredient should be whole wheat flour, brown rice, rye flour, oats, or barley. Enriched wheat flour is refined grain with nutrients added back. Enriched products include all- purpose flour, cake flour, bleached flour, bread flour, white rice, and white pasta.

- **Sugar:** This is a simple or fast acting carbohydrate and include the following:
    1. Naturally occurring sugars including lactose (milk sugar) and fructose (fruit sugar).
    4. Sugars that are added in processing such as baking, syrups and canned fruit syrup. Common processed sugar names include table sugar, powdered sugar, brown sugar, high fructose corn syrup, molasses, honey, confectioner's sugar, and maple syrup.

Quick tip

Avoid or restrict processed sugars as much possible. All of these products will have a high glycemic index which allows a rapid fluxuation of the serum glucose (blood sugar level). This allows glucose to be driven into the cells and be converted into fat.

- **Fiber:** This is derived from plant foods and the non digestible part of fruits, vegetables, legumes, whole grains, and nuts. There is no fiber in meat, fish, chicken and poultry, milk, and eggs. Adults need to ingest 25-30 grams of fiber per day and most fiber passes through the intestines without being digested. Total fiber is the combination of dietary fiber and functional fiber. Fiber is divided into two categories:

1. Soluble fiber: Dissolves in water to a gel like substance. Excellent sources include fruits such as apples/bananas/berries, some vegetables, psyllium, oats, and legumes.
2. Insoluble fiber: Does not dissolve in water. Sources include whole wheat products, nuts, seeds, bran, and some vegetables and fruits (particularly the skin).

Quick tip

Both soluble and insoluble fibers are beneficial. Fiber is effective in gastrointestinal disorders (such as Irritable Bowel Syndrome), lowering cholesterol, controlling weight, and lowering serum glucose (helping to prevent and control diabetes).

- **Simple ways to increase fiber intake:**
    1. Multiple vegetable servings daily
    2. Fresh vegetables cut up as snacks
    3. Cereal with higher fiber content
    4. Products with whole wheat flour (or whole wheat grains)
    5. Add legumes such as peas and beans to any dish when possible
    6. Add frozen berries to cereal, shakes, or yogurt
    7. Add flaxseeds, nuts, and seeds to any dish when possible

Fats

- **Monounsaturated fatty acid (MUFA):** This includes oleic acid (main fat in olive oil) and palmitoleic acid and is an excellent fat with minimal down side. MUFA help decrease fatty deposits in vascular walls by decreasing the oxidation of LDL. (Oxidized LDL has a greater propensity to stick to the walls of the arteries and therefore increases the risks of heart attacks and strokes). Olive oil may also increase fat burning rather than promoting fat storage. Exercise help to burn MUFA's and therefore decreases fat storage. Overall, appropriate total fat (including MUFA) should comprise 20-30% of your daily caloric intake. **MUFA sources include olive oil, peanut oil, canola oil, olives, avocadoes, nuts (peanuts, almonds, and macadamias).**

Quick tip

Substitute Olive oil (or other MUFA) when possible, careful with excessive saturated fats, and eliminate all trans fat.

- **Polyunsaturated fatty acids (PUFA):** This includes linoleic acid (omega-6), alpha-linoleic acid (ALA/ omega-3), eicosapentaenoic acid (EPA/ omega-3), docosahexaenoic acid (DHA/ omega-3), and conjugated linoleic acid (CLA). Interesting facts on PUFA:
    1. **Omega- 6:** These are essential fatty acids that must be consumed in a food source as they cannot be produced by the body. In general we eat too many Omega-6 fatty acids (added to multiple foods) as compared to Omega-3. The optimum ratio for Omega-6 to Omega-3 is 3:1. Too high an intake of Omega-6 may result in excessive inflammation in the body and this may predispose to cardiac disease, arthritis, obesity, and cancer. **Sources of Omega-6 include soybean oil, corn oil, sunflower oil, and sesame oil.**
    2. **Omega-3:** The two types that are particularly important are EPA and DHA and it is extremely important to supplement these in a diet. Omega-3 fatty acids help prevent heart disease, lower triglycerides (and to some degree cholesterol levels), help control obesity, have anti-inflammatory effects (joints, blood vessels, and organs), improve glucose metabolism, and may

have antidepressant effects. Omega-3's also increase fat burning and lower total body fat. **Excellent sources of Omega-3 include cold water fish (white tuna, salmon, herring, sardines, mackerel, and trout), flaxseed, walnuts, mayonnaise, soft margarine, and omega enriched eggs.**

3. **Conjugated linoleic acid:** CLA improves muscle mass and inhibits fat deposition. These are found in red meat and dairy products.

Quick tip

Monounsaturated fats are more heat stable and are better to cook with as compared to polyunsaturated fats.

- **Saturated fats:** Include palmitic acid (dairy), stearic acid (beef and chicken), and lauric acid (coconut). Generally the goal is to keep saturated fats at a minimum and consume only the saturated fats found naturally in food sources such as meat, dairy products, and eggs. We clearly need to avoid the saturated fats found in baked goods, processed foods, and lard as there are minimal positive effects. Saturated fat consumption becomes a major problem when you are simultaneously consuming excess carbs and excess calories as there is additional oxidation of LDL. This oxidized LDL deposits in the walls of blood vessels and predisposes to heart attacks and strokes. These are many potential benefits to saturated fats that are obtained through dietary sources. With the appropriate carb and calorie intake, the saturated fats are less likely elevate cholesterol and may actually improve the HDL (good cholesterol) to LDL (bad cholesterol) ratio. This decreases the risks of heart attack and stroke. Dietary saturated fat also helps to improve testosterone production and helps improve muscle mass. **Sources include beef, chicken, pork, dairy, lard, and coconut oil.**

Quick tip

Saturated fats found in natural food products may elevate the good cholesterol (HDL) and improve the Triglyceride to HDL ratio and LDL to HDL ratio. This can be beneficial and is the basis for the recommendation to insure the saturated fat intake is obtained through dietary sources.

- **Trans and Esterified fat:** This includes vegetable oils that have been hydrogenated to solid fat. The bottom line is that trans fat improves food taste but is extremely unhealthy. Try to avoid all trans fat intake. **Sources include shortening, fried foods, hydrogenated margarine, crackers, packaged pastries and cookies.**

Best Food Winners

This section lists by category the foods with the best nutritional value. The great part of this food list is that all of these foods also have excellent taste value, particularly when seasoned and cooked appropriately. Remember that these are the best, but there are many other extremely nutritious choices. The final section in this chapter lists the best fast food choices with an emphasis on Subway as this is clearly the best overall option in this category. Be careful with the serving size as this will affect the overall calories, but there is no need to specifically count calories. Remember that we typically underestimate caloric intake so add 25% to your count to obtain a reasonable true estimate. Caloric breakdowns are provided here for reference purposes so you can start learning how to estimate the amount you are consuming.

Meat and Fish Protein: 3-4oz servings

- **Chicken Breast**: Skinless- 140cal/3.1grams fat/0.9grams saturated fat. This meat is the staple of a healthy diet.
- **Turkey breast**: Skinless- 161cal/4grams fat. Another excellent protein source equivalent to the chicken breast.
- **Orange Roughy**: 75cal/0.8grams fat/0grams saturated fat. Orange roughy has the lowest fat content of all fish. **Tilapia** is also an excellent inexpensive choice.
- **Salmon**: 175cal/11grams fat/2.1grams saturated fat- particularly high in Omega 3. This is an excellent fish protein stable for any healthy diet.
- **Top Sirloin**: 156cal/4.9grams fat/1.9grams saturated fat. This steak provides a red meat option with reasonable fat content. Beef is bred to increase fat marbling (Kobe beef is a prime example) and this extra fat content improves the taste. Unfortunately this also dramatically decreases the healthy nutritional value of the meat. Top sirloin has excellent taste with a reasonable fat content.

Quick tip

Oily/cold water fish such as salmon, herring, tuna, halibut, and sardines are high in Omega 3. The correct Omega 6 to Omega 3 ratio decreases inflammation. Extra Omega 3 intake in our diet or in supplements is very beneficial as our normal diet is generally low in this nutrient.

Dairy/Eggs/Cheese

- **Egg whites**: Eggs overall are ranked as the best single protein food source and contain all of the essential amino acids.
- **Whole eggs**: The American Heart Association recommends a maximum of one egg per day. The white portion contains the protein but the yolk does have excellent nutritional benefit. When scrambling eggs have one whole egg to maximize taste and then add additional egg whites for the protein.
- **Skim/Nonfat milk**: An excellent source of calcium, protein, and vitamins.

Fruits

- **Berries**: Strawberries, blueberries, and raspberries are all low calorie, high fiber, low carbs, no fat, with excellent antioxidants and phytochemicals.
- **Citrus**: Orange, grapefruit, and Clementine's are low calorie (15-80 calories), low to medium carbs, excellent folate, potassium, B6, thiamine, niacin, and Vitamin C, no fat, with excellent phytochemicals and antioxidants.
- **Melons**: Cantelope and Honeydew are low calorie, low carbs, excellent vitamin A, excellent vitamin C, and no fat.
- The fantastic nutritional value of fruits should always be emphasized.

Quick tip

For maximum carbohydrate use, concentrate fruit intake in the first half of the day and try to avoid fruits in the evening. Vegetable carbs can be consumed any time during the day and should be the primary source of carbs in the evening.

Vegetables

- **Broccoli**: Low calorie, minimal carbs, excellent vitamin A and C, potassium, riboflavin, calcium, iron, excellent phytochemicals and antioxidants, and no fat. This is clearly the best food in the vegetable and fruit category.
- **Spinach**: Low calorie, minimal carbs, excellent vitamin A, C, and E, excellent B carotene, calcium, iron, fiber, potassium, excellent phytochemicals and antioxidants, and no fat.
- **Tomato**: Low calorie, minimal carbs, excellent potassium, vitamin A and C, Iron, excellent antioxidants and phytochemicals and no fat. Tomatoes have a high lycopene content which may decrease the risk of various types of cancer. They are actually botanically a fruit but are used as a vegetable.
- **Asparagus**: Low calorie, minimal carbs, excellent vitamin A, B6, folate, iron, calcium, excellent antioxidants and phytochemicals, and no fat.
- Vegetables are equal to fruits in nutritional value and should be emphasized in a healthy diet.

Quick tip

Single best fruit or vegetable is broccoli with tomatoes a close second.

Nuts: 1oz serving

- **Almonds**: 169 calories/6grams protein/5grams carbs/15grams fat- excellent fat burning with antioxidants and Omega 3. Currently the most advertised healthy nut.
- **Walnuts**: 185 calories/4grams protein/4grams carbs/18grams fat- an excellent antioxidant with Omega 3.
- **Pecans**: Contain the highest antioxidant levels of the nut family.
- **Pistachios**: Excellent taste with high antioxidants and Omega 3 content.
- **Peanut butter:** This is always an important part of all healthy diets. It is important to watch for peanut butter allergies as this reaction can be fatal. Most people will learn during childhood if this is a problem.
- Nuts are a fantastic source of protein but have a high salt content. The best option is unsalted nuts although from my perspective there is a taste loss.

Bread/Rice

- **Whole wheat pita**
- **Wild Rice**
- **Quinoa:** This little known grain contains all of the essential amino acids with a healthy dose of unsaturated fats and less carbohydrates than rice or bread. It can be precooked and stored in the refrigerator. Quinoa has a flavorful nutty taste and can be substituted for rice or other grains in many recipes.

Quick tip

Whole wheat bread, Sourdough, Pumpernickel, and Rye are excellent bread choices. "Cracked wheat" or multigrain breads are not better than whole wheat.

Cereal

- **Regular Oatmeal:** Top with banana, berries (blueberries, raspberries, or strawberries), or walnuts for extra nutrition.
- **Instant Oatmeal:** Sugar free or low sugar is the optimal choice. Many instant oatmeal products will contain high fructose corn syrup. HFCS is added for taste but the intake should be minimized as this promotes the deposition of fat.

Fast Food: Remember that fast food is never the first choice in a healthy diet. Generally you should attempt to restrict the number of times per week that you are eating fast foods. Certain choices at Subway are the exception, but remember not all options at Subway are healthy.

- **Subway:** 6 inch Turkey or Ham with multiple vegetables – 210 calories/13grams protein/36grams carbs/3.5grams fat/1.5grams saturated fat/730mg sodium. Subway clearly leads the rest of the fast food category in nutritional value. When you are pressed for time, go to Subway and order healthy.
- **Taco Bell:** Taco Supreme Fresco Style – 150 calories.
- **Pizza Hut:** Fit and Delicious Pizza, one slice: Ham/Red onion/Mushroom – 150 calories/8grams protein/21grams carbs/4grams fat/2grams saturated fat/440mg sodium OR Green pepper/Red onion/Tomatoes – 140 calories/6grams protein/22grams carbs/4grams fat/1.5grams saturated fat/330mg sodium.
- **McDonalds:** Grilled Chicken Salad with Newman's low fat Balsamic – 240 calories/29grams protein/13grams carbs/9grams fat/3grams saturated fat/1550mg sodium.
- **Arby's:** Hot Ham and Swiss Melt – 270 calories/18grams protein/35grams carbs/8grams fat/4grams saturated fat/1140mg sodium. Ask for tomatoes

and lettuce to be added to the sandwich for extra nutrition without significant extra calories.

- **Chick-fil-A:** Chargrilled Chicken Sandwich- 270 calories/3.5grams fat/1gram saturated fat/940mg sodium.
- **Quiznos:** Small Honey Bourbon Chicken on wheat bread- 310 calories/4grams fat/1gram saturated fat/920mg sodium.
- **Schlotzsky's:** Small Smoked Turkey Breast Sandwich- 345 calories/5grams fat/1240mg sodium.
- The fast food industry is constantly changing their menu and responding to the higher demand for healthy options. It is helpful to consult the web sites of the various fast food restaurants and evaluate the nutritional content of new options. If the restaurant does not provide the nutritional breakdown, there is a high probability they are hiding information and you should be suspicious of any nutritional claims made by that company.

Fruit Nutritional Information

Brief Review: alphabetical order

- **Apples**: higher carbs, excellent fiber and phytochemicals
- **Avocado**: higher fat but healthy unsaturated fat, excellent fiber, vitamins, phytochemicals, folate
- **Banana**: medium carbs, excellent fiber, vitamin C, potassium
- **Berries**: blueberry/raspberry/strawberry/cranberry- low carb, high fiber, excellent phytochemicals and antioxidants
- **Citrus**: orange/grapefruit/clementine- variable carbs, excellent fiber, vitamin C, B vitamins, excellent phytochemicals and antioxidants
- **Grapes**: red/green- medium carbs, excellent vitamin C, potassium, excellent phytochemicals
- **Melons**: cantaloupe/honeydew- low carbs, excellent vitamin A and C, fast digestion, excellent phytochemicals- watermelon with medium carbs
- **Pears**: medium carbs, excellent fiber, vitamins, minerals, excellent phytochemicals
- **Stone fruit**: apricots/cherries/peach/prunes/plums- low to medium carbs, excellent fiber, vitamin C, B vitamins, excellent phytochemicals and antioxidants
- **Tropical fruit**: mango- excellent vitamins A, C, D- papaya- excellent fiber, folate, vitamin A, papain
- **Pineapple**: excellent vitamin C, folate, iron, B vitamins, fiber

Quick tip

Fruits are best consumed earlier in the day with vegetable carbohydrates any time but particularly later in the day. Some fruits do have a higher glycemic index but generally are extremely healthy. Even with a high glycemic index the fruit may have a lower glycemic load (example: watermelon).

Vegetable Nutritional Information

Brief Review: Alphabetical order: most are low calorie, low carb with no fat

- **Asparagus:** Excellent source of Vitamin A, B6, folate, iron, and calcium with excellent phytochemicals and antioxidants.
- **Broccoli:** Overall broccoli is the best vegetable or fruit: Very nutrient dense with excellent potassium, Vitamin A, Vitamin C, riboflavin, calcium, iron with excellent phytochemicals and antioxidants.
- **Brussels sprouts:** Excellent source of Vitamin A, Vitamin C, fiber, calcium, and iron with excellent phytochemicals and antioxidants.
- **Cabbages:** Excellent source of fiber, folate, calcium, iron, Vitamin K, potassium, and Vitamin C with excellent phytochemicals.
- **Carrots:** Excellent source of Vitamin A, calcium, and iron but with moderate carbohydrates.

Quick tip

Salads with fresh vegetables added are an excellent staple of the healthy diet. Broccoli, Spinach, Carrots, Zucchini, Mushrooms, Onions, Peppers, Cauliflower, and Cucumbers are all excellent additions. Cabbage or spinach mixed with lettuce is very nutritious. Legumes such as Chick peas, green beans, and peas add excellent protein and nutrition to the salad.

- **Cauliflower:** Creates full feeling quickly which makes this an excellent food to control or lose weight. Cabbage is an excellent source of Vitamin C, iron, and calcium.
- **Corn:** Excellent source of Vitamin A, Vitamin C, iron, protein, potassium, and fiber.
- **Cucumbers:** Excellent source of Vitamin A, Vitamin C, and potassium.
- **Greens: Spinach:** Excellent source of Vitamin A, Vitamin C, Vitamin E, calcium, Beta carotene, iron, fiber, and potassium with excellent antioxidants.

- **Green Lettuce**: Excellent source of Vitamin A, Vitamin C, calcium, and iron.
- **Legumes**: Includes multiple different beans and peas with variable calories depending on the specific type. All types are excellent source of protein, folate, fiber, and potassium.

Quick tip

Legumes are particularly high in protein and are crucial parts of all diets, but mandatory in vegetarian diets. Vegetarians must be careful to combine different sources of protein to insure that all essential amino acids are covered in their diet.

- **Mushrooms**: Different mushrooms have variable calories, although the most popular types are generally low calorie with excellent sources of B vitamins, selenium, potassium, and copper.
- **Onions**: May be dry or fresh green all with excellent levels of vitamin C, potassium, folate, and iron. All types are excellent sources of antioxidants.
- **Peppers**: Include both sweet and chili: All types are excellent sources of Vitamin A, Vitamin C, Vitamin E, potassium, folate, iron, calcium, and B vitamins.
- **Potato with skin**: Contain moderate carbs, but excellent fiber, Vitamin C, potassium, B6, and minerals.
- **Tomato**: Excellent source of potassium, Vitamin A, Vitamin C, and iron with excellent phytochemicals and antioxidants (lycopene).
- **Zucchini**: Quickly creates a full feeling making this a very helpful weight loss or weight maintaining food. Zucchini is an excellent source of Vitamin A, Vitamin C, and potassium.

Quick tip

Broccoli is the single best vegetable or fruit, but tomatoes are excellent also - particularly with the high lycopene levels.

Monthly Nutritional Shopping List

The goal is to establish good eating habits and this starts with cooking at home and learning to cook the correct, nutritious meals. By planning the week in advance you can be efficient, know what you are eating each day, and not succumb to the urge to eat out after a tough day at work. The stocked items should be kept in the pantry at all times and then there is a weekly breakdown of what to purchase in order to fix the meals that are outlined in the weekly menu's that follow this chapter. Remember to evaluate the menu before you go shopping and change any meal that you would not enjoy. Also consider the leftover food before shopping each week in order to prevent food wastage. Each weekly shopping list is designed to feed one person.

Stocked items: These items form the foundation of your kitchen.

Condiments/Herbs:

- Mustard- simple yellow or fancy if you prefer
- Ketchup- high fructose corn syrup free is the optimal choice
- Black pepper grinder
- Sea salt grinder- or regular iodized salt
- Garlic powder
- Onion powder
- Basil- dried
- Oregano- dried
- Pepper blend (McCormick)- a personal favorite
- Parsley- dried
- Chili powder
- Cumin- dried/powder
- Crushed Red pepper
- Rosemary- dried
- Thyme- dried
- Minced garlic

> **Quick tip**
>
> Herbs add excellent flavor without adding unnecessary calories.

Dressings:

- Low fat Balsamic Vinaigrette dressing (Newman's is my favorite)
- Low fat Red wine Vinaigrette dressing (Newman's)
- Low fat Caesar dressing (Newman's)
- Low fat Raspberry dressing (Newman's)
- Fat free Ranch dressing (Hidden Valley)
- Low fat Miracle whip
- Low fat Olive oil based butter or margarine
- Extra virgin Olive oil
- Balsamic vinegar

Sauces and Broths:

- Low sodium Chicken broth- Swanson's has excellent and taste and is cost efficient
- Low sodium Soy sauce- Kikoman's is the best
- Low calorie/low fat Maple syrup
- BBQ Sauce- excellent flavor and low calorie
- Marinara sauce- Bertoli's is my favorite- can use for spaghetti or flat bread pizza

Drinks:

- V8 juice- 4oz cans for portability (great for snacks)
- Orange juice with calcium
- Apple juice- cloudy is the best choice as it contains the most nutritional value
- Skim milk

Nut products:

- Almonds
- Smooth peanut butter

Quick tip

Low fat peanut butter simply elevates the simple sugar content so go with the good tasting regular peanut butter. The full feeling achieved from a small amount of peanut butter will prevent you from eating excess calories. Also this is an excellent source of protein.

Cereal and Breakfast bars:

- Special K breakfast bars (or South Beach bars or personal choice). Of note Special K bars do not have any HFCS
- Cereal: Multigrain Cheerios, Special K, Total, etc- your choice but do not choose a cereal with a high glycemic index
- Oatmeal
- Low fat Granola

Dairy and egg products:

- Low fat Mozzarella cheese sticks (Sargento is my favorite)
- Low fat American cheese slices
- Low fat Jarlsberg cheese slices (excellent taste with lower fat)
- Low fat Parmesan cheese
- Eggs- high Omega 3, range free
- Egg beaters

Canned/frozen fruits:

- Applesauce- no sugar added individual servings

- Low fat Mixed fruit- individual servings
- Four berry frozen fruit mixture

Frozen vegetables:

- Frozen Broccoli
- Frozen Mixed Vegetables
- Frozen Green Beans
- Frozen Peas

Bread or bakery items:

- Whole wheat bread
- Whole wheat flat bread- can be used for flatbread pizza or as a wrap
- Trisket crackers

Canned Salsa

- Salsa- mild, medium or hot (your preference)- may also make this fresh

Frozen, preserved, or canned Meat/Fish products:

- Shrimp bag- frozen
- Precooked Chicken strips- frozen
- Healthy Choice or Lean Cuisine frozen dinners- stock a variety of different meals
- Turkey pepperoni
- Tuna- water packed

Quick tip

Substitute fish, shrimp, soy crumbles, or vegetable burger if you do not eat meat.

Week One Shopping List- based on one person

Fresh items:

- Bananas- 2
- Apples- 2
- Clementine's- 1
- Strawberries- 1 small container
- Red seedless Grapes
- Grape tomatoes- 1 small container
- Cantaloupe- 1 whole
- Cucumber- 1
- Green onions- 1 bunch
- Red onion- 1
- Zucchini- 1, small
- Beefsteak tomato- 1
- Green bell pepper- 1
- Celery hearts- 1 bag
- Baby Carrots- 1 bag
- Asparagus- 1 small bunch
- Mushrooms- 4
- Sweet Onion- 1
- Jalapeno pepper- 1
- Russet potato- 1
- Romaine lettuce- 1 bunch

Quick tip

To improve the overall flavor of asparagus, snap off the woody bottom part before cooking.

Canned goods:

- Red kidney beans- 15 ½ oz can
- Crushed Tomatoes- 28 oz can

Chip items:

- Pretzels- 1 bag

Dairy products:

- Yogurt- Light and Lively- 3 French vanilla
- Low fat Feta cheese- small package
- Sour cream- fat free- 8 oz

Bread and bakery:

- Whole wheat Bagel- 1
- Whole wheat Hamburger buns- 1 package

Meat and Fish products:

- Center cut bacon or Turkey bacon- small package
- Top Sirloin- 6 oz
- Chicken breast- 6 oz
- Low fat Hamburger- 10 oz (may substitute Vege burgers for the hamburger and Soy protein/Vegetable crumbles in the chili)
- Orange Roughy- 6 oz (may need to find this in the frozen section)—a secondary option is Tilapia- 6 oz

Quick tip

Remember to factor in left over's from last week when you are shopping for the next week.

Week Two Shopping List

Fresh items:

- Bananas- 4
- Strawberries- 1 small container
- Red seedless grapes
- Pineapple squares
- Lemon- 1
- Apples- 2- type is your choice but gala and fuji are very sweet
- Green onions- 1 bunch
- Cucumber- 1
- Mushrooms- 4
- Celery hearts- 1 bunch
- Baby carrots- 1 bag
- Spinach- 1 bag
- Red onion- 1
- Sweet onion- 1
- Red bell pepper- 1
- Zucchini- 1, small
- Grape tomatoes- 1 small container
- Asparagus- 1 small bunch
- Romaine lettuce- 1 bunch

Dairy products:

- Yogurt- Light and Fit- 2 French vanilla

Canned items:

- Petite diced tomatoes- one 12 oz can

Bread and bakery

- Whole wheat English muffins
- Whole wheat rolls- small package

Meat and Fish products:

- Low fat Hamburger- 6 oz (or Vegetable burgers)
- Chicken breasts- Two 6 oz
- Pork loin- 6 oz
- Sea scallops- 4 large

Quick tip

Pure Pork loin will not have any additives listed on the label.

Week Three Shopping List

Fresh items:

- Bananas- 4
- Strawberries- 1 small package
- Red seedless grapes- medium bunch
- Cantaloupe- 1
- Honeydew- 1
- Apple- 1
- Lemon- 1
- Lime- 1
- Sweet onion- 1
- Red onion- 1
- Celery hearts- 1 bunch
- Baby carrots- 1 bag
- Red bell pepper- 1
- Portobello mushroom- 1 small package
- Mushrooms- 4
- Corn on the cob- 2 ears
- Grape tomatoes- 1 small container

- Jalapeno pepper- 1
- Green onion- 2 bunches
- Romaine lettuce- 1 head
- Boston lettuce- 1 head
- Cilantro- fresh- 1 bunch
- Asparagus- 1 small bunch
- Zucchini- 1, small
- Yellow squash- 1, small

Canned items:

- Petite diced tomatoes- two 12 oz cans
- Navy beans- 15 oz can

Chip items:

- Pretzels- 1 bag

Bread and bakery:

- Whole wheat rolls – 1 small package

Cereal items:

- Special K Protein snack bar- 2

Dairy products:

- Fat free Sour cream- 8 oz container
- Yogurt- Light and Fit- French vanilla 3 small containers
- Low fat shredded Mozzarella cheese- 8 oz package

Meat and Fish items:

- Top Sirloin- 6 oz
- Snow Crab legs- ½ lb
- Wild Salmon- 6 oz- wild has a higher Omega 3 content as compared to farm raised

Week Four Shopping List

Fresh items:

- Bananas-4
- Cantaloupe- 1
- Red grapes
- Grape tomatoes- 1 small container
- Baby carrots- 1 small package
- Celery hearts- 1 bunch
- Green onions- 2 bunches
- Red onion- 1
- Sweet onion- 1
- Asparagus- 1 bunch
- Red bell pepper- 1
- Beefsteak tomato- 1
- Boston lettuce- 1 head
- Romaine lettuce- 1 head
- Red potatoes- 1
- Mushrooms- 2
- Corn on the cob- 1

Dairy products:

- Light and Fit yogurt- 2 small French vanilla
- Pesto sauce- premade- usually near the refrigerated cheeses

Canned goods:

- Bertoli's marinara sauce- 1 (if not already in stock)

Bread and bakery:

- Whole wheat English muffins- 1 package
- Whole wheat pitas- 1 package
- Whole wheat pasta- 1 package
- Whole wheat rolls- 1 small package

Meat and Fish products:

- Chicken breast- 6 oz
- Top sirloin- 6 oz
- Cooked lump crab meat- 8 oz- find in the refrigerated section near the fresh seafood

- Low fat Hamburger- 6 oz
- Sea scallops- 4
- Wild salmon- 6 oz

Quick tip

Any left over's from last week-- change the menu to use them up.

Healthy Nutrition: Week 1

Week 1	Monday	Tuesday	Wednesday	Thursday	Friday	Saturday	Sunday
Breakfast	Cheerios with sliced banana 6oz skim milk 4oz coffee	½ Whole wheat English muffin toasted topped with peanut butter and sliced apples 6oz Orange Juice (OJ)	Egg beater scrambled with veges and low fat cheese 1 slice ww toast	Breakfast bar Light and Lively Yogurt 6oz AJ (Apple Juice)	Cheerios with sliced strawberries 6oz skim milk	2 Fried Eggs Center cut bacon 1 sliced ww toast 6oz OJ	Smoothie with one banana, strawberries, OJ, and ½ whole wheat English muffin
Snack	Celery, Carrots, Grape Tomatoes	4oz V8 Juice Pretzels	Light and Fit Yogurt with low fat granola 1oz Almonds	Light string cheese 1 cup red grapes	4oz V8 Juice Trisket crackers	Clementine Trisket crackers	Hard boiled egg Grape Tomatoes
Lunch	Tuna fish wrap Pretzels 1 cup red grapes	Subway 6 inch Baked chips	Turkey sandwich with low fat Jarsberg Cubed cantaloupe Pretzels	Frozen dinner Cubed cantaloupe	Restaurant Grilled chicken wrap Steamed Broccoli	Grilled cheese with tomato 1 cup Applesauce Pretzels	Chicken or Shrimp Tortilla Roll 1 cup low fat Mixed Fruit
Snack	Clementine orange Trisket crackers	1 cup Applesauce 1oz Almonds	Light string cheese 1 cup red grapes	Hard Boiled egg Grape tomatoes	Celery with peanut butter	4oz V8 Juice Pretzels	1 cup grapes 1oz Almonds
Dinner	Grilled Chicken 6oz Broccoli Tomato/Onion and Mozzarella cheese side salad	Grilled Cheeseburger Grilled Asparagus Grilled Onion Banana	Chopped Dinner Salad with Shrimp ½ ww Bagel with butter and garlic then broiled	Orange Roughy 6oz Green beans Sliced Tomato side salad	Spaghetti with Marinara sauce Broccoli Caesar side salad	Top Sirloin 6oz Baked potato Broccoli Chopped side salad	Chili Whole Wheat Roll

Healthy Nutrition: Week 2

Week 2	Monday	Tuesday	Wednesday	Thursday	Friday	Saturday	Sunday
Breakfast	Cheerios with sliced banana 6oz skim milk	Breakfast bar Light and Lively Yogurt with low fat granola 6oz skim milk	1 Fried egg Center cut bacon 1 slice ww English muffin 6oz OJ	Oatmeal with 1tsp low fat butter 1 slice whole wheat toast	Smoothie- banana with strawberries, OJ, and yogurt	Egg English Muffin with low fat cheese 1 banana 6oz OJ	Low fat Pancakes with low fat Maple syrup Turkey bacon 6oz skim milk
Snack	4oz V8 Juice Pretzels	Celery with peanut butter	Light string cheese 1 cup red grapes	Hard boiled egg 1 cup applesauce	Celery, Carrots, Grape Tomatoes	4oz V8 Juice Trisket crackers	Light and Fit Yogurt- with low fat granola Trisket crackers
Lunch	Turkey or Ham wrap Cubed Cantaloupe	Frozen dinner 1 cup red grapes	Subway 6 inch Baked chips	Tuna wrap 1 cup grapes Pretzels	Restaurant low fat salad Fruit side dish	BBQ Chicken Pita Cubed Cantaloupe	Vege/Cheese wrap Strawberries and banana sliced Pretzels
Snack	Turkey pepperoni Low fat Fruit cup	Light string cheese 1oz Almonds	4oz V8 Juice Pretzels	Clementine orange Wheat thins	Turkey pepperoni Hard Boiled Egg	Celery, Carrots, and Grape Tomatoes	Apple slices Trisket crackers
Dinner	Grilled Pork loin 6oz with BBQ sauce Green beans Romaine side salad Whole wheat roll	Sea Scallops with spinach Tomato/onion and cubed mozzarella side salad Broccoli ½ ww English muffin	Grilled Hamburger with chopped onion and spinach Chopped salad Grilled zucchini Grilled Onion	Grilled Chicken 6oz Grilled Asparagus Grilled Red Pepper Whole Wheat Roll	Apple Lettuce Salad Toasted whole wheat English muffin	Shish Kebob with chicken and shrimp Applesauce cup	Vegetable Soup Dinner Chopped side salad Whole wheat roll

Healthy Nutrition: Week 3

Week 3	Monday	Tuesday	Wednesday	Thursday	Friday	Saturday	Sunday
Breakfast	Oatmeal with 1tsp low fat butter 1 slice ww English muffin 6oz skim milk	Scrambled egg beater with veges 1 slice ww English muffin 6oz OJ	Cheerios with sliced banana 6oz OJ	Smoothie with banana, strawberries, OJ, yogurt	Oatmeal with sliced bananas 6oz skim milk	Cheerios with sliced strawberries 6oz AJ	Egg tortilla with fresh salsa 6oz OJ
Snack	Strawberries 1 low fat string cheese	Light fruit cup	Light and Fit Yogurt with low fat granola	1 cup applesauce 1oz Almonds	Special K snack bar	Light and Fit Yogurt with low fat granola	Low fat Jarlsberg Trisket crackers
Lunch	Tuna fish wrap Cubed Cantaloupe and Honeydew	Subway 6 inch Baked chips	Frozen dinner Light fruit cup	Low fat Ham wrap Cubed Cantaloupe and Honeydew	Subway 6 inch Baked chips	Chopped side salad with precooked chicken	Frozen dinner One cup red grapes
Snack	Baby carrots, celery, grape tomatoes	4oz V8 Juice Pretzels	Special K snack bar	Turkey pepperoni Trisket crackers	1oz Almonds Hard boiled egg	4oz V8 Juice Pretzels	Apple slices
Dinner	Baked Chicken Breast 6oz Roasted Veges Whole wheat roll	Grilled Salmon 6oz Grilled Asparagus and grilled Onions Boston lettuce chopped side salad	BBQ Flatbread Pizza Boston lettuce chopped side salad Applesauce cup	Grilled Chicken 6oz topped with fresh salsa Broccoli Caesar side salad	Steamed Snow Crab Legs Corn on the cob Broccoli Whole wheat roll	Steak (top sirloin) and Portobella mushroom fajitas Corn on the cob	Navy Bean soup with Grilled Cheese and tomato Banana sliced with peanut butter

Healthy Nutrition: Week 4

Week 4	Monday	Tuesday	Wednesday	Thursday	Friday	Saturday	Sunday
Breakfast	Smoothie Banana and four berries with OJ and low fat yogurt	Cheerios with sliced banana 6oz OJ	Egg on ww English muffin and slice low fat cheese 6oz AJ	Oatmeal with sliced bananas 6oz skim milk	Cheerios ½ ww English muffin 6oz AJ	Egg Tortilla 6oz skim milk	Low fat Pancakes with sliced bananas and applesauce Center cut bacon 6oz AJ
Snack	Celery, Carrots, Grape tomatoes	4oz V8 Juice Pretzels	Light fruit cup	Light and Fit Yogurt with low fat granola	1cup Applesauce 1oz Almonds	Clementine orange Trisket crackers	String cheese Grape Tomatoes
Lunch	Tuna fish pita 1cup red grapes	Turkey pita Cubed Cantaloupe	Frozen dinner Light fruit cup	Subway 6 inch Baked chips	Vege/cheese wrap Pretzels	Grilled cheese with tomato 1cup Applesauce	BBQ chicken pita Cubed Cantaloupe
Snack	Lite Jarlsberg cheese Trisket crackers	Hard boiled egg 1oz Almonds	Clementine orange 1 String cheese	4oz V8Juice Pretzels	Turkey pepperoni Trisket crackers	Celery, Carrots, Grape Tomatoes	4oz V8 Juice Pretzels
Dinner	Grilled Chicken 6oz Broccoli Side salad Grilled Sliced Red Onion	Grilled Salmon Grilled 6oz Asparagus Grilled Red Bell Pepper Whole wheat roll	Baked Sea Scallops with onion, carrots, red bell pepper Caesar side salad	Chicken Soup Dinner Sliced Beefsteak Tomato Whole wheat roll	Spaghetti Broccoli Whole wheat roll	Maryland Crab Cakes Chopped side salad Green beans	Top Sirloin 6oz Corn on the cob Grilled Asparagus Whole wheat roll

Monthly Exercise Regimen

Exercise is a crucial part of health and wellness. When embarking on an exercise regiment, be sure you are medically cleared by your primary physician or a cardiologist. People who have been sedentary or have a high risk of cardiac disease may require a cardiac stress test to insure there are no hidden heart problems. When starting on the program the key is to start slow and increase your activity on a weekly basis and don't forget to warm up before each session. The following outlines suggested monthly programs for:

- ✓ **Novice level**
- ✓ **Intermediate level**
- ✓ **Advanced level**

***Remember all exercises can be done at home or in a health club. Exercising with a friend is always very beneficial but make sure you and your friend are approximately the same goals.

Aerobic exercise options: The monthly outline will establish specific exercise recommendations but you are free to adjust to any of these aerobic suggestions. When using a computer program on an exercise machine, choose a lower level and slowly increase the resistance as your fitness improves. Also change the program on a monthly basis as this will prevent you from reaching a plateau which will prevent further gain. If the program offers interval training, this is an excellent option.

- Semi-recumbent bike: This is an excellent baseline aerobic exercise as there is minimal strain on the hips, knees, and ankles, and can be done while watching TV or reading.
- Outdoor biking: Great aerobic work out with enjoyable scenery. Men in particular need to be cautious with pressure from the seat on the perineal area as this may cause erectile problems.
- Treadmill: Indoor equivalent of running. Use the interval training portion of the program to improve the exercise regimen.

- Running: The ultimate aerobic exercise although high stress levels on the hips, knees, and ankles.
- Fast walking: Make sure it is fast and not a leisurely stroll.
- Elliptical machine: Essentially equal to running with less stress on the hips, knees, and ankles.
- Rowing machine: Excellent aerobic exercise which allows simultaneous work of the lower and upper body.
- Stairmaster: Fantastic work out but stressful to the knees and hips. People with underlying lower joint problems should avoid this machine.
- Swimming: Provides high quality aerobic exercise with upper and lower body work out. Swimming should be the first choice of people with arthritic problems as the water will help suspend your joints and prevent excess stress.
- Jumping rope: This takes time to learn, but provides aerobic exercise with upper and lower body work out and coordination training.
- Inline skating: Excellent aerobic exercise but wear appropriate protection with at least head gear and wristgards. Chose a path that is smooth without excessive pot holes or gravel/rocks.
- Athletic event: The correct athletic competitive events are great from an aerobic standpoint and enjoyable.

Quick tip

Running, treadmill, and elliptical are all interchangeable excellent aerobic exercises. My personal favorite is the semi recumbent bike followed by a short work out on the elliptical machine. Add interval sets weekly to prevent a plateau.

Aerobic Interval Sets: Intervals help significantly with participation in athletic events and are also an excellent fat burning technique.

- **Interval Set #1:** 50 meter sprint with 15 second rest in between reps. One set is 5 sprints. Can also be done on the treadmill.
- **Interval Set #2:** 50 meter sprint with 15 second rest in between reps. One set is 10 sprints. Can also be done on the treadmill.
- **Interval Set #3:** 100 meter sprint with 15 second rest in between reps. One set is 5 sprints. Can also be done on the treadmill.
- **Interval Set #4:** 100 meter sprint with 15 second rest in between reps. One set is 10 sprints. Can also be done on the treadmill.
- **Interval Set #5:** 200 meter sprint on the bike, ride slowly for 15 seconds, and repeat the sprint. One set is 5 sprints. Can also be done on the semi recumbent bike.
- **Interval Set #6:** 200 meter sprint on the bike, ride slowly for 15 seconds, and repeat the sprint. One set is 10 sprints. Can also be done on the semi recumbent bike.
- **Interval Set #7:** 25 meter sprint in the pool with 15 second rest in between reps. One set is 5 sprints.
- **Interval Set #8:** 25 meter sprint in the pool with 15 second rest in between reps. One set is 10 sprints.
- **Interval Set #9:** 50 meter sprint in the pool with 15 second rest in between reps. One set is 5 sprints.
- **Interval Set #10:** 50 meter sprint in the pool with 15 second rest in between reps. One set is 10 sprints.

Anaerobic (Weight lifting) options: Buy a book or obtain appropriate training in the use of this equipment in order to optimize your exercise results and prevent injury.

- Dumbbells: Inexpensive weight set which can be used in many different ways.
- Free weights: It is important to use a spotter to decrease the injury potential.
- Weight machines: Many excellent machines are available in a health club setting or for home purchase.
- Swiss ball: Great to use alone or in combination with dumbbells.

Weight lifting sets: Start with the weight which suits your strength level and then slowly increase the weights as your strength increases. The correct weight should tire you at the end of the set. Sets generally consist of 8, 10, or 15 reps. The 8 rep set uses heavier weights and is best for muscle mass formation. The 10 rep set should be a slightly less weight and is beneficial for muscle mass formation and for muscle definition. 15 rep sets are the lowest weight and are primarily for muscle definition. All three levels of weight lifting are important and should be done with the intermediate and advanced levels. When in the novice phase it is more important to develop a consistent regimen that you will maintain so stay with the 10 rep set.

- **Set 1:** Done with dumbbells. Consider buying a book with descriptions and pictures of dumbbell exercises or take one or two lessons from a personal trainer. Incorrectly done exercises can result in injury.
  - Bicep curls: Do both arms at the same time. With arms hanging at your side and palms facing outward from the front of your body, curl the weight up to your bicep. Then slowly let the weight back down.
  - Brachialis curls: Same as the bicep curls except change your hand orientation to the palm facing the outside of your leg.
  - Triceps press: Dumbbell held above your head with the elbow bent. Then extend your arms to the ceiling.
  - Deltoid fly's: Dumbbell at your side with your palm pointed toward the outside of your thigh. Then extend both arms sideways and upward away from your body.
  - Military press: Dumbbells held above your head with elbows bent and palms pointed inward toward the head. Then directly extend your arms toward the ceiling.
  - Pectoralis curls on Swiss ball: Lie on the Swiss ball with the small of your back and have your arms with the dumbbells directly out from your side. Then curls both dumbbells back to above the center of your chest.
  - Pushups on Swiss ball: With feet on the Swiss ball do pushups. The will also help with the abdominal muscles.

> Sit-ups on Swiss ball: Lie on the Swiss ball with the small of your back and do sit ups. Always take your time both up and down and do not "rock" on the ball.

- **Set 2:** Once you have reached the intermediate or advanced phase you should either be quite comfortable with the different types of exercises, or you should take at least one lesson from a personal trainer. Incorrectly done exercises can cause injury.
    > Dumbbell curls
    > Dumbbell brachialis curls
    > Machine triceps push down
    > Machine pectoralis curls
    > Machine military press
    > Machine bench press
    > Dumbbell deltoid fly's
    > Machine quad presses
    > Machine hamstring curls
    > Gastroc presses
    > Pushups on Swiss ball
    > Sit-ups on Swiss ball

Quick tip

Remember to change your regimen approximately once a month. This will prevent plateau's where your fitness level dose not continue to improve. In down times where you do not feel like working out be sure to push for exercise sessions 1-2 times per week. This will prevent a regression in your fitness level.

Novice Exercise Regimen

Sunday	Monday	Tuesday	Wednesday	Thursday	Friday	Saturday
AM: Aerobic: Semi bike 10 minutes PM: Aerobic: Semi bike 10 minutes Weights: Set #1 with 5 reps & 1 set	Off	AM: Aerobic: Semi bike 10 minutes PM: Aerobic: Running 5 minutes Weights: Set #1 with 5 reps & 1 set	Off	AM: Aerobic: Semi bike 10 minutes PM: Aerobic semi bike 10 minutes Weights: Set #1 with 5 reps & 1 set	Off	AM: Aerobic: Interval set #1 Weights: 10 push ups
AM: Aerobic: Semi bike 15 minutes PM: Aerobic: Semi bike 15 minutes Weights: Set #1 with 8 reps & 2 sets	Off	AM: Aerobic: Semi bike 15 minutes PM: Aerobic: Running 5 minutes Weights: Set #1 with 8 reps & 2 sets	Off	AM: Aerobic: Semi bike 15 minutes PM: Aerobic: Semi bike 15 minutes Weights: Set #1 with 8 reps & 2 sets	Off	AM: Aerobic: Interval set #1 Weights: 15 push ups
AM: Aerobic: Running 7 minutes PM: Aerobic: Semi bike 20 minutes Weights: Set #1 with 10 reps & 2 sets	Off	AM: Aerobic: Semi bike 20 minutes PM: Aerobic: Semi bike 10 minutes Weights: Set #1 with 10 reps & 2 sets	Off	AM: Aerobic: Semi bike 30 minutes PM: Aerobic: Semi bike 5 minutes Weights: Set #1 with 10 reps & 2 sets	Off	AM: Aerobic: Interval set #3 Weights: 20 push ups
AM: Aerobic: Semi bike 30 minutes PM: Aerobic: Semi bike 5 minutes Weights: Set #1 with 10 reps & 2 sets	Off	AM: Aerobic Semi bike 30 minutes PM: Aerobic: Semi bike 5 minutes Weights: Set #1 with 10 reps & 2 sets	Off	AM: Aerobic: Running 10 minutes PM: Aerobic: Semi bike 5 minutes Weights: Set #1 with 10 reps & 2 sets	Off	AM: Aerobic: Interval set #3 Weights: 20 push ups

Intermediate Exercise Regimen

Sunday	Monday	Tuesday	Wednesday	Thursday	Friday	Saturday
AM: Aerobic: Semi bike for 30 minutes PM: Aerobic: Semi bike for 15 minutes Weights: Set #2 with 8 reps & 2 sets	Off	AM: Aerobic: Running for 20 minutes PM: Aerobic: Semi bike for 25 minutes Weights: Set #2 with 8 reps & 2 sets	AM: Aerobic: Semi bike for 45 minutes PM: Aerobic: Semi bike for 10 minutes Weights: Set #2 with 10 reps & 2 sets	Off	AM: Aerobic: Semi bike for 45 minutes Weights: Set #2 with 10 reps & 2 sets	AM: Aerobic: Interval set #1 Weights: 20 push ups PM: Aerobic: Semi bike for 30 minutes
AM: Aerobic: Semi bike for 30 minutes PM: Aerobic: Semi bike 30 minutes Weights: Set #2 with 10 reps & 3	Off	AM: Aerobic: Semi bike for 30 minutes PM: Aerobic: Semi bike for 15 minutes Weights: Set #2 with 15 reps & 3 sets	AM: Aerobic: Running for 20 minutes PM: Aerobic: Semi bike for 25 minutes Weights: Set #2 with 10 reps & 3 sets	Off	AM: Aerobic: Semi bike for 45 minutes Weights: Set #2 with 15 reps & 3 sets	AM: Aerobic: Interval set #5 Weights: 20 push ups PM: Aerobic: Semi bike for 30 minutes
AM: Aerobic: Semi bike for 30 minutes PM: Aerobic: Semi bike for 30 minutes Weights: Set #2 with 10 reps & 3 sets	Off	AM: Aerobic: Running for 20 minutes PM: Aerobic: Semi bike for 30 minutes Weights: Set #2 with 8 reps & 3 sets	AM: Aerobic: Semi bike for 45 minutes PM: Aerobic: Semi bike for 10 minutes Weights: Set #2 with 15 reps & 3sets	Off	AM: Aerobic: Semi bike for 45 minutes Weights: Set #2 with 10 reps & 3 sets	AM: Aerobic: Interval set #2 Weights: 30 push ups PM: Aerobic: Semi bike for 30 minutes
AM: Aerobic: Semi bike for 30 minutes PM: Aerobic: Semi bike for 30 minutes Weights: Set #2 with 10 reps & 3 sets	Off	AM: Aerobic: Semi bike for 45 minutes PM: Aerobic: Semi bike for 10 minutes Weights: Set #2 with 8 reps & 3 sets	AM: Aerobic: Running for 20 minutes PM: Aerobic: Semi bike for 30 minutes Weights: Set #2 with 15 reps & 3 sets	Off	AM: Aerobic: Semi bike for 45 minutes Weights: Set #2 with 10 reps & 3 sets	AM: Aerobic: Interval set #6 Weights: 30 push ups PM: Aerobic: Semi bike for 30 minutes

Intermediate Exercise Regimen

Intermediate Exercise Regimen for the Time Impaired

Sunday	Monday	Tuesday	Wednesday	Thursday	Friday	Saturday
AM: Aerobic: Semi bike for 40 minutes / Weights: Set #2 with 10 reps & 3 sets / PM: Aerobic: Running for 20 minutes	Off	AM: Aerobic: Interval #3 / Weights: Set #2 with 10 reps & 3 sets	AM: Aerobic: Semi bike for 45 minutes / Weights: Set #2 with 10 reps & 3 sets / PM: Aerobic: Running for 15 minutes	Off	AM: Aerobic: Semi bike for 60 minutes / Weights: Set #2 with 10 reps & 3 sets	AM: Aerobic: Interval set #1 / Weights: 20 push ups
AM: Aerobic: Semi bike for 40 minutes / Weights: Set #2 with 8 reps & 4 sets / PM: Aerobic: Running for 20 minutes	Off	AM: Aerobic: Interval #5 / Weights: Set #2 with 10 reps & 4 sets	AM: Aerobic: Semi bike for 45 minutes / Weights: Set #2 with 15 reps & 4 sets / PM: Aerobic: Running for 15 minutes	Off	AM: Aerobic: Semi bike for 60 minutes / Weights: Set #2 with 10 reps & 4 sets	AM: Aerobic: Interval set #5 / Weights: 20 push ups
AM: Aerobic: Semi bike for 40 minutes / Weights: Set #2 with 8 reps & 4 sets / PM: Aerobic: Running for 20 minutes	Off	AM: Aerobic: Interval #4 / Weights: Set #2 with 10 reps & 4 sets	AM: Aerobic: Semi bike for 45 minutes / Weights: Set #2 with 15 reps and 4 sets / PM: Aerobic: Running for 15 minutes	Off	AM: Aerobic: Semi bike for 60 minutes / Weights: Set #2 with 10 reps & 4 sets	AM: Aerobic: Interval set #2 / Weights: 30 push ups
AM: Aerobic: Semi bike for 40 minutes / Weights: Set #2 with 8 reps & 4 sets / PM: Aerobic: Running for 20 minutes	Off	AM: Aerobic: Interval #6 / Weights: Set #2 with 10 reps & 4 sets	AM: Aerobic: Semi bike for 45 minutes / Weights: Set #2 with 15 reps and 4 sets / PM: Aerobic: Running for 15 minutes	Off	AM: Aerobic: Semi bike for 60 minutes / Weights: Set #2 with 10 reps & 4 sets	AM: Aerobic: Interval set #6 / Weights: 30 push ups

Advanced Exercise Regimen

Sunday	Monday	Tuesday	Wednesday	Thursday	Friday	Saturday
AM: Aerobic: Semi bike for 40 minutes / Weights: Set #2 with 8 reps & 3 sets / PM: Aerobic: Running for 20 minutes	AM: Aerobic: Semi bike for 40 minutes / PM: Aerobic: Running for 20 minutes / Weights: Set #2 with 10 reps & 3 sets	Off	AM: Aerobic: Semi bike for 30 minutes / PM: Aerobic: Semi bike for 30 minutes / Weights: Set #2 with 15 reps & 3 sets	AM: Aerobic: Running for 20 minutes / PM: Aerobic: Semi bike for 40 minutes / Weights: Set #2 with 10 reps & 3 sets	Off	AM: Aerobic: Interval set #3 / Weights: Set #2 with 10 reps & 3 sets / PM: Aerobic: Semi bike for 30 minutes
AM: Aerobic: Semi bike for 40 minutes / Weights: Set #2 with 8 reps & 4 sets / PM: Aerobic: Running for 20 minutes	AM: Aerobic: Semi bike for 40 minutes / PM: Aerobic: Running for 20 minutes / Weights: Set #2 with 10 reps & 4 sets	AM: Aerobic: Semi bike for 30 minutes / PM: Aerobic: Semi bike for 30 minutes / Weights: Set #2 with 15 reps & 4 sets	Off	AM: Aerobic: Running for 20 minutes / PM: Aerobic: Semi bike for 40 minutes / Weights: Set #2 with 8 reps & 4 sets	AM: Aerobic: Semi bike for 60 minutes / Weights: Set #2 with 10 reps & 4 sets	AM: Aerobic: Interval set #5 / Weights: Set #2 with 15 reps & 4 sets / PM: Aerobic: Semi bike for 30 minutes
AM: Aerobic: Semi bike for 40 minutes / Weights: Set #2 with 8 reps and 4 sets / PM: Aerobic: Running for 20 minutes	AM: Aerobic: Semi bike for 40 minutes / PM: Aerobic: Running for 20 minutes / Weights: Set #2 with 10 reps & 4 sets	AM: Aerobic: Semi bike for 30 minutes / PM: Aerobic: Semi bike for 30 minutes / Weights: Set #2 with 15 reps & 4 sets	Off	AM: Aerobic: Running for 20 minutes / PM: Aerobic: Semi bike for 40 minutes / Weights: Set #2 with 8 reps & 4 sets	AM: Aerobic: Semi bike for 60 minutes / Weights: Set #2 with 10 reps and 4 sets	AM: Aerobic: Interval set #4 / Weights: Set #2 with 15 reps & 4 sets / PM: Aerobic: Semi bike for 30 minutes
AM: Aerobic: Semi bike for 40 minutes / Weights: Set #2 with 8 reps and 4 sets / PM: Aerobic: Running for 20 minutes	AM: Aerobic: Semi bike for 40 minutes / PM: Aerobic: Running for 20 minutes / Weights: Set #2 with 10 reps & 4 sets	AM: Aerobic: Semi bike for 30 minutes / PM: Aerobic: Semi bike for 30 minutes / Weights: Set #2 with 15 reps & 4 sets	Off	AM: Aerobic: Running for 20 minutes / PM: Aerobic: Semi bike for 40 minutes / Weights: Set #2 with 8 reps & 4 sets	AM: Aerobic: Semi bike for 60 minutes / Weights: Set #2 with 10 reps & 4 sets	AM: Aerobic: Interval set #6 / Weights: Set #2 with 15 reps & 4 sets / PM: Aerobic: Semi bike for 30 minutes

Part II

Exercise

Exercise

Exercise and nutrition form the two major building blocks of wellness. A fit, toned physique permits optimal cardiovascular and lung function along with preventing or assisting in controlling multiple medical and metabolic problems. Even if you are de-conditioned now, exercise can restore your body's fitness level and improve your sense of well being. The key is to start slow and progressively improve your fitness. Once you reach your goal never let it go again. You will appreciate how you feel now, and will clearly be ahead as the year's progress.

Quick tip

Before starting an exercise program, insure adequate medical clearance first. This initial medical exam is extremely important as you do not want to embark on an exercise regiment if there are underlying medical problems which should be adequately treated and controlled.

Exercise pearls:

- **Aerobic exercise:** This form of exercise should be done 3-4 times per week with 20-45 minutes per session. Daily sessions can be split into shorter periods in the morning and evening, but it is crucial to exercise hard each time. For the most efficient weight loss, 5-6 times per week becomes imperative. It is important for wellness to maintain cardiovascular fitness.
- **Anaerobic exercise:** Weight lifting should be done 2-4 times per week as it is imperative to optimize your muscle tone. This will also help with fat burning as your body will switch to an aerobic phase for 8-12 hours after the weight lifting session. Women do not need to worry about developing excessive muscle bulk as this requires heavy lifting for an

extended period of time. The lower testosterone level found in women will prevent the development of bulky muscles.

- **Exercise session timing:** The optimum is to complete the daily work out in one continuous time frame. If this is not possible with your schedule, there is excellent data to show that breaking up the sessions in two or even three 10-20 minute sessions in a given day is equally efficient. The key is to maximize your effort with each session.

- **Warm up and Cool down:** Before each exercise session, warm up with brisk walking, slow running, lower level elliptical, lower level stairmaster, low speed biking, or swimming. This warm up phase is crucial to prevent injuries. After the session, cool down with similar activities or simply slow down what ever exercise you are doing. This cool down phase should last for 5-10 minutes and then you should complete your exercise session with stretching. The warm up and cool down times do not count towards your recommended exercise time.

- **Stretching:** This is best done daily in the early AM and is equally important after exercise sessions. Stretching **does not** replace the warm up and cool down periods.

- **Optimize:** Insure that every workout counts by exerting yourself at 90-100% effort each session. This becomes even more important if you are breaking your sessions into multiple shorter intervals over the course of the day.

- **Change:** Vary your exercise regiment once a month otherwise your results will plateau. Consider varying your aerobic exercises within the same work out, again to prevent boredom. As an example: Use the elliptical and stationary bike and split the time.

- **Recovery:** Give your body a chance to recover and rebuild the muscle. Do not lift weights on a daily basis that involve the same muscle group. It is very important to completely take off one day per week. You must let your body heal and rebuild.

- **Realistic:** Set goals that you can reach, both aerobically and from a weight lifting standpoint. Once you reach your goals pick new ones or vary your routine to maintain a high level of fitness.

- **Work out diary:** Keep a log of each exercise, weight used, repetitions, number of sets, and aerobic exercise time. This will assist in pushing you to new levels.

- **Down time:** Everyone will go through periods of time when their exercise motivation level is low. One full work out per week will prevent you from regressing in your fitness level. Try to resume your regular exercise regiment within 2 weeks.

- **Companion work out:** Most people will be more efficient working out with a friend. Make sure both of you have similar fitness goals and similar abilities in the gym. This will provide optimum results with the exercise sessions.
- **Nutrition:** This is always extremely important. A "6 pack ab" cannot be achieved with sit ups and aerobic exercise only. This is truly a nutrition first situation with exercise an important second.
- **Fluids:** Stay hydrated before, during, and after the session with plenty of fluid intake.
- **Carbohydrate loading:** It is important to insure adequate carbohydrate intake before and after exercise sessions. Exercise will deplete the glycogen in your muscles and you must reload this glycogen with adequate carbohydrate intake. The harder the session or activity, the more carbohydrates you will need before and after.

Quick tip

With **aerobic exercise** your muscles are using oxygen on a continuous basis during the session. This increases heart and lung capacity. Generally this is with exercises such as brisk walking, running, biking, swimming, etc. **Anaerobic exercise** is associated with weight lifting or very intense activity. During this time your muscles are functioning with the oxygen that was already present within the muscle tissue. After completion of the anaerobic exercise, your muscles will convert back to an aerobic metabolism and replenish their oxygen supply.

Warm up and Cool down

- **Warm up:** This is extremely important overall. It involves 5-10 minutes of lower level aerobic activity which sets the tone for the work out and promotes the appropriate blood flow to muscles, lungs, and heart. When the muscles are ready for the session there is a lower risk of injury. The warm up also allows the heart rate to increase in a controlled fashion and decreases the risk of adverse cardiac events. Warm up options include:

1. Brisk walk
2. Light jogging
3. Slow paced bike riding
4. Low level elliptical or stairmaster
5. Slow paced swimming

- **Cool down:** Essentially the reverse of the warm up phase. If you are doing an aerobic exercise at the completion of your work out, simply slow down the intensity of this exercise but if you are weight lifting change to an aerobic exercise as listed in the warm up section. Cooling down will allow the heart rate and muscle blood flow to return in a gradual fashion to their normal level.

Stretching

Daily stretching of tendons and muscles promotes the flexibility of joints. This decreases injury risk and promotes good posture. **Rules of stretching** include:

- **Daily:** Stretch daily in the AM. This will help maintain appropriate muscle balance between opposing muscle groups.
- **After:** Stretch after the cool down phase of each work out. Data suggests that at the beginning of exercise sessions it is more important to warm up than stretch.
- **Slowly:** Slow stretching movements are the key. Never jerk or snap yourself into a position and never bounce once you are in a position.
- **Relax:** Allow your muscles to be in a relaxed mode and try not to contract them during the stretch. Completely relax the muscle group in between stretches.
- **Tension:** Slowly take the muscle into a position of mild tension all the way up to severe tension. Do not try to produce sharp pain as this could result in muscle or tendon tears.
- **Hold:** Once in position, hold for 2 deep breaths in order to obtain maximum effect.
- **Progressive:** Slowly increase your flexibility over several weeks and then strive to maintain the flexibility. Optimal flexibility cannot be achieved in one session.

Basic stretching: work from top to bottom.

1. **Neck:** Gently rotate your head in a 360 degree pattern. Rotate clockwise and counterclockwise. Then use your right hand to pull the head to the right and then your left hand to pull your head to the left. Keep your shoulders relaxed during the maneuvers.

2. **Chest:** Hold your arms out to the side and gently rotate 360 degrees in small circles. Then bring your arms behind your back, clasp them together, and gently lift your arms toward the ceiling.

3. **Back:** Hold your arms out in front at chest height, clasp your hands, and stretch your back into a C shape.

4. **Lateral torso:** Use a straight bar held across your shoulders behind your neck. Put your hands on either end of the bar and rotate your torso from side to side.

5. **Quadriceps:** While standing, grab your right foot with your right hand and pull your foot up behind you and stretch your right quad. Repeat with your left hand and left leg.

6. **Hamstrings:** While sitting with your legs straight out reach out with your hands and touch your toes. Try not to bend your knees to any significant degree. Hamstrings are a common athletic injury due to the difficulty in adequately stretching this muscle group therefore it is important to pay attention to the hamstrings.

7. **Calf:** Standing facing a wall reach out with your hands and lean into the wall. Then gently lean your chest into the wall to stretch the calf muscles.

8. **Groin:** In a butterfly sitting position slowly push your knees downward with your forearms.

Quick tip

Remember to slowly stretch the muscle group and then hold for 2 breaths. If you are experiencing any sharp pain, the stretching is too far.

Indoor Aerobic Exercise

1. **Treadmill:** This machine may used for a hard walk or for running. Treadmill programs allow for varying the speed and incline during the work out. As with running, treadmills may cause extra stress on ankles, knees, and hips, but provide a high quality indoor aerobic session. Be careful to start slowly and use the automatic shut off mode in case you lose your balance. Look forward and do not hold onto the handrails.

2. **Cycling:** Options for indoor cycling include the semi recumbent and upright bikes. My preference is clearly the semi recumbent bike. This bike has a broader based seat with the pedals out in front of you and allows less strain on the knees, lower back, and perineal area. The upright bike provides the same aerobic exercise and enthusiasts of this bike feel it is a better simulation of outdoor cycling. Programs permit variation in speed and resistance for more variety. **Spinning** is a special indoor bike generally used at a health club in a class format. The class format helps to increase motivation.

3. **Elliptical:** This machine has broad foot pads and is a mixture of cross country skiing, fast walking or running, and stair climbing. The arm motion build into the machine motion adds to the total caloric burn on these machines. This is truly an excellent work out without the stress on knees and ankles and is my second favorite indoor exercise. It is very difficult to read on the elliptical machine so plan on another form of distraction such as a favorite TV show or sporting event.

4. **Stair climber/Stair Master:** Another excellent aerobic work out similar to running stairs outside. The stair machine does result in significant strain on the knees and also can be very difficult for people just starting their exercise routine. This machine is for the more advanced exercise enthusiast.

5. **Rowing machine:** If this is done correctly, it is an excellent work out for legs, arms, and chest in addition to the aerobic component. Remember that the motion starts from the legs.

6. **Jumping rope:** This is a superb exercise which involves multiple muscle groups simultaneously with a hard aerobic component. It is a favorite of boxers but is an extremely beneficial component of any exercise

regiment. Add it to your regiment to promote variety. The coordination involved in jumping rope may take time to learn so be patient.

Quick tip

Don't forget to vary your aerobic activity to prevent boredom. Also try and insure that you have appropriate distractions (scenery, reading, TV, etc) so you are not simply "watching the clock." Exercise is mentally painful if you are counting the seconds.

Outdoor Aerobic Exercise

1. **Walking and Running/Jogging:** Running and jogging are clearly the bench marks for aerobic conditioning. If walking is done it must be high energy (walking fast) for an appropriate aerobic benefit. Combinations of walking and running can also be very effective particularly during the times when you are trying to increase your cardio fitness.
    Running/Jogging results in a higher stress level on the ankles, knees, and hips than many other forms of exercise. People with underlying injuries to their hips, knees, ankles, or feet may find that this increases their chronic discomfort. It is very important to have comfortable running shoes with appropriate cushion.

2. **Bicycling:** This is an excellent aerobic exercise with less strain on the ankles, knees, and hips. It is also fun as you can cover large distances and observe the scenery which helps prevent boredom. Caution must be used if riding in areas where cars may be present due to the risk of injury. Obviously bike trails are the optimum, but are hard to find. Men in particular need to be very careful with the pressure the seat on an upright bike applies to the perineum (the area between your anus and scrotum) as this pressure can potentially have long term neurological effects

including impotence. It is important to intermittently stand while riding to relieve this pressure. Head injuries are also a major concern with cycling so wear a helmet!!!

3.   **Swimming:** This is also an excellent aerobic exercise with minimal pressure on the joints. It can be boring as there is no scenery, so try and focus on the comfort of the water as this can be very soothing psychologically. You may also run in the pool or do pool aerobic classes if your swimming technique is suboptimal. Pool weights are available which can be used to intensify the work out.

4.   **In-Line Skating/Rollerblading:** These techniques are high quality aerobic exercises which simultaneously work multiple muscle groups. They can be fun as you cover large distances with different scenery. Injuries are common as it can be difficult to change directions and stop quickly. Particularly worrisome injuries are to the head and wrist therefore it is important to wear a helmet and wrist guards. As with biking, be careful when cars may be present as they increase the injury risk. Trails are clearly the optimum place to inline skate. Watch for rocks, gravel, holes in the pavement, etc. as it will take time to learn how to change direction quickly.

5.   **Cross Country Skiing:** Many experts believe this is the best combination of aerobic exercise and muscle group work out. There is no question this is a great work out. When done in the mountains, cross country skiing can be coupled with fantastic scenery. This is a great way to work out in the winter when you live in a cold, snowy climate. With any outdoor winter activity, make sure you dress appropriately and don't forget to wear sunscreen and appropriate eye cover. Sunburn and corneal burns are common in snowy conditions.

6.   **Snowshoeing:** This is another excellent outdoor winter activity with high quality aerobic results. Overall an inexpensive way to enjoy the outdoors and beautiful scenery while you are working out. Make sure you learn on packed trails as you will be surprised how difficult snowshoeing can be in fresh deep snow.

7.   **Hiking:** Inexpensive, enjoyable high quality aerobic exercise. Choose the right hike and take your camera for great pictures to enjoy later. Make sure you pick a trail that corresponds to your fitness level and invest in good quality hiking shoes. Don't forget to take sufficient water and snacks particularly if you are hiking in the wilderness.

8.   **Mountain biking:** Another great outdoor aerobic activity with excellent scenery. This does require a moderate investment in a good mountain bike with appropriate tires and springs. It is crucial to wear a helmet.

Athletic activities: Aerobic exercise can also be derived from a competitive sports activity, both individual and team oriented. Join a team or participate from an individual standpoint, then substitute this activity on game day for your regular aerobic activity.

1.   **Basketball:** Full court BB is an excellent aerobic exercise. Half court pick up basketball can also be as good an aerobic event as long as there are not too many breaks.

2.   **Soccer:** Join a league and play full field soccer or consider a smaller field 8 a side. Both are equally aerobic. Of note, high level soccer players are considered the second fittest athlete in all of sports. Interestingly, motocross is number one.

3.   **Tennis:** Single's tennis with minimal breaks is an excellent aerobic activity.

4.   **Racquetball:** Fantastic aerobic exercise.

5.   **Golf:** Great exercise if you walk and carry your bag. Riding in a cart does not count.

6.   **Skiing, Snowboarding, Cross Country Skiing, and Snowshoeing:** High quality aerobic exercise particularly if you save the time in front of the fire for the end of the day.

7.   **Kayaking:** Both sea and whitewater kayaking are equally superb.

Weight lifting

Major reasons to weight lift:

1.   **Metabolism:** During the actual weight lifting period your muscles are generally functioning in an anaerobic state. Once the weight lifting session is over your muscles change to a prolonged aerobic state which may last 8-12 hours. During this time your metabolism is running at higher speeds and fat burning will occur without any additional exercise.

2. **Health:** Excellent muscle tone promotes a healthy skeletal system including bones and associated tendons and ligaments. As age moves on, weight lifting will help prevent bone loss (osteoporosis), and helps delay the normal loss of muscle mass.

3. **Vanity:** Clearly strong, toned muscles look good. Feeling good about "you" is a part of overall health and wellness.

4. **Psychological:** In addition to feeling good about how you look, exercise and weight lifting will promote the release from the brain of a chemical called endorphins. Endorphins promote mental wellness and an overall feeling of satisfaction.

5. **Injuries:** Healthy, toned muscles lower the risks of injury with athletic endeavors and also with the activity of daily living. Excellent muscle tone is particularly important for the "weekend athlete." Remember, we all need to get to work on Monday!!

Quick tip

Reps (Repetition) are the number of consecutive times you complete one full motion of a particular exercise. The most common number of reps in a set is 8, 10, 12, and 15.

Sets (or Set) are the number of reps in a group of a particular exercise. For example one set may include 10 reps and you may do 2 or 3 sets of a given exercise.

Pearls of weight lifting:

- Start slow and build up the reps and sets that you do during one weight lifting session.
- Don't forget to warm up and cool down.

- Take your time during one rep and remember to breathe. 2 seconds up and at least 2 seconds down is very reasonable. Use a full range of motion for each rep.
- Each muscle group generally should have 2-4 sets per weight session. 30 seconds between sets is a reasonable resting period. When using heavier weights consider a lesser number of sets, and with lighter weights increase the sets per session.
- Do not work the same muscle groups on consecutive days. Your muscles need time to heal.
- For muscle bulk use higher weights and lower reps such as 8 per session. The last rep should be difficult to complete or you need to use more weight.
- For muscle tone and definition use lower weights and higher reps such as 12-15 per session.
- Best option is to vary the weight and repetitions from session to session. This will insure that you adequately work all of the different muscle fibers.
- Your muscles need to be fatigued at the end of the sessions for maximum effect on muscle tone and growth.
- Weight lifting sessions should be done 2-4 times per week. For maximum effect work out different muscle groups on different days and lift 5-6 times per week.
- Always have one full day off per week from all exercise. Give your body a fair chance to repair itself.
- Change your routine once a month. If you are doing the same exercise and weight lifting routine for long periods you will plateau and become frustrated with the lack of improvement.
- Learn to lift correctly and with appropriate form. This will decrease the injury risk.
- Remember that abdominal muscle tone (the 6 pack) is nutrition first with aerobic exercise and weights an important second.
- When in a slump and having a hard time motivating yourself to work out, as a minimum lift weights once a week. This will generally prevent your gains from slipping backwards.
- Weight lift with a friend to help motivate each other and push to new exercise heights.
- Free weights versus Machine weights: Both are good and have their advantages and disadvantages. Free weights work more muscle groups at one time as you need to maintain the balance of the weights. The

injury risk is higher with free weights and when pushing yourself you should have a spotter. Machine weights generally work on the muscle group it is designed for and have a lower injury rate. Beginners should use the machines and add free weights in later as their strength and conditioning improves.

- Circuit training: Can be very beneficial as it is set up to provide a reasonable overall body weight lifting experience.

Muscle Groups

1. **Upper Body:**
   - **Shoulder-** Deltoids/Rotator cuff
   - **Back-** Trapezius/Latissimus dorsi/Rhomboids/Erector spinae
   - **Chest-** Pectoralis major and minor
   - **Arms-** Biceps/Triceps/Forearm muscles
   - **Abdominals-** Rectus abdominis/Internal and External obliques
2. **Lower Body:**
   - **Buttocks and Hips-** Gluteus maximus and minimus/Hip abductors/Leg adductors
   - **Legs-** Quadriceps/Hamstrings/Gastrocnemius/Soleus/Tibialis anterior

Weight lifting options

- **Dumbbells and Swiss Ball:** These are inexpensive, effective, and my favorite simple gym. The dumbbell sets do not have to be fancy and the Swiss ball allows multiple exercises with and without weights. You can have a full gym for less than $100. An excellent source for types of sets to be done is found in the Swiss Ball Core Workout by Declan Condron, Sterling publishing.
- **Machine work out:** This generally involves the use of cable based machines. There are many different varieties of machines and different price ranges that are available for home purchase. Weight lifting

machines are safe and easy to use. Make sure the weight stack meets your overall needs.

- **Free weights:** There are weight sets which are quite economical and available for home use. Spend a small amount extra for the clips to hold the weights on as this will save time when changing the weights on the bar. Buy the basic set and add individual weights as you need them. Weight lifting requires balance during the exercise rep and should be done with a spotter to help prevent injuries.

- **Health club:** All good health clubs will have a combination of free weights and machines so you can mix and match to improve your weight session and prevent boredom. Clubs will be expensive over time, but can also be fun with different equipment available to vary your exercise sessions. Additionally, training partners and personal trainers are easily available. Personal trainers certainly help with learning the correct weight lifting technique and also by pushing you to new levels. The best choice is a certified personal trainer who will tailor the work outs to your personal needs and abilities. Take the time to research the trainer who will best serve your needs or you will end up wasting money. To be cost effective alternate your sessions; one with the trainer and one without.

- **Travel bands:** Buy a set to take on trips and combine with push ups for an "on the road" weight lifting session. Dumbbells are also available for travel. Simply add water to the plastic dumbbell to create the weight.

Part III

Nutrition

Nutrition and Diet Introduction

Nutrition is one of the primary foundations of a healthy lifestyle and wellness. A person's diet helps prevent disease by providing the appropriate building blocks which allow your body to fight the onset of disease. Additionally these same nutritional keys will assist your body in the repair process needed for the treatment of illness. Each person needs to individualize their diet to fit their lifestyle and optimize their health.

Nutritional tips:

- **Eating patterns:** Clearly the most important point in dietary modulation. Eating small amounts frequently over the course of the day prevents rapid fluxuations in the blood insulin levels. Rapid elevations in the insulin will drive glucose into the cells and allow this to be converted to fat. The optimum diet is 5-6 small meals per day which maintains a relatively steady level of blood glucose. This includes breakfast, mid morning snack, lunch, mid afternoon snack, dinner, and potentially a very small evening snack. If possible the evening snack should include casein protein (milk protein) which is a long acting protein which promotes muscle repair over the course of the night.

- **Moderation and Variety:** Vary the diet from meal to meal and day to day to maintain interest and insure a healthy intake of different nutrients. Initially keep a **food diary** where you write down all of the food you eat daily and then roughly calculate your total caloric intake. This diary will help provide you with a more accurate reading of how much you are truly eating. If a food diary is not used then remember we generally underestimate how many calories we eat per day so always add 25% to the number of calories that you believe were consumed. Review your diet frequently to prevent you from slipping into an overeating or unhealthy food intake pattern.

- **Carbohydrates:** Not necessary low carbs but it very important to eat the correct carbs. The correct carbs include whole wheat grain products, fruits, and vegetables/legumes. Whole wheat products should replace refined grains such a white bread and white pasta. Concentrate the fruit and grain intake in the first 2/3 of the day for the most part and vegetables all day with an emphasis at dinner.

- **Protein:** Lean protein is the key. This includes beef with the fat trimmed off (particularly top sirloin), chicken and turkey (white meat without the skin), low fat hamburger (or Maverick beef), pork (particularly pork tenderloin), fish, center cut or turkey bacon, scallops, and shrimp (although slightly higher in cholesterol). Legumes such as beans and peas are also excellent protein sources.

- **Fat:** Unsaturated fats are the best. Monounsaturated fats (olive and canola oil), and polyunsaturated fats including Omega-3 (cold water fish, walnuts, almonds) and Omega-6 (foods made with soy, peanut, and corn oil) are clearly the optimum. Our diet is high in Omega-6 and we need to concentrate on increasing the intake of Omega-3. Attempt to minimize the saturated fat intake to the more healthy variety found in meat, fish, dairy, and eggs. Completely avoid trans fat and esterified fat intake.

- **Processed foods:** Avoid or minimize food with hidden sugar intake. This is very prevalent in fast foods and processed foods.

- **Alcohol and Regular Soda:** Essentially empty calories and should be avoided.

- **Caffeine:** Acceptable in small amounts daily.

- **Fluid:** Water intake is particularly important for optimum health.

- **Gradual improvement:** Sudden, large changes in lifestyle are generally not successful. It is best is to adjust your diet and exercise pattern slowly and attempt to make the change over a 2-3 month period. It is then crucial to maintain the change on a daily basis.

- **Cheat day/meal:** Once you are stable in your new lifestyle and are at the weight you are comfortable with, add a cheat "day". This is **one meal** per week where you may eat what you want. The cheat meal will help prevent breaking down and eating unhealthy foods on other days as you mentally will know that for the "Friday dinner" you may have whatever you are craving.

Quick tip:

5-6 small meals per day is the most important alteration to your diet which will improve your overall health and wellness.

Antioxidants and Phytochemicals

Antioxidants and phytochemicals are substances which help remove dangerous byproducts (free radicals) generated by the body. The removal of these compounds decreases the inflammatory changes in the body and decreases the risk of cancer. In general the supplementation of these antioxidants has not been shown to be as beneficial as obtaining these materials from food products. The following is a short look at the current known antioxidants and phytochemicals along with representation foods that contain these compounds.

Antioxidants

These are chemicals which remove free radicals and therefore decrease cancer risk and inflammation. Current antioxidants include the following:

- **B Carotene**
- **Vitamin A**
- **Vitamin C**
- **Vitamin E**
- **Selenium**
- **Molybdium**
- **Alpha-Lipoic Acid (ALA)**
- **Manganese**
- **Zinc**
- **Copper**

Phytochemicals

These are plant related antioxidants that remove free radicals. These chemicals decrease cancer risk and inflammation. Additionally, phytochemicals decrease allergies, lower total cholesterol and LDL (both of which block arteries), and balance estrogen metabolism. They may decrease heart disease, decrease fluid retention, and decrease diabetic neuropathy. Current phytochemicals include the following:

- **Flavonoids**: Broccoli, garlic, onions, carrots, peppers, cabbage, grapes.
- **Carotenoids**: Sprouts.
- **Lycopene**: Tomatoes, soy.

- **Indoles**: Broccoli, Brussel sprouts, cabbage.
- **Capsaicin**: Tomatoes, red grapefruit, watermelon.
- **Phytosterols**: Citrus.
- **Genistein**: Soybeans, peas, cabbage.
- **Sulfroraphane**: Broccoli, chili peppers.
- **Allium**: Strawberries.

Vitamins and Minerals

Vitamins

Vitamins are micronutrients that the body ingests and uses without breaking them down. Fat soluble vitamins include A, D, E, and K. Excessive intake of fat soluble vitamins can cause a buildup of a specific vitamin in the body and potentially harmful effects. Water soluble vitamins include C and the eight B vitamins. Any excess of these vitamins will be cleared by the body and buildup does not occur. In general, people with a normal diet will still commonly be deficient in folic acid, B6, B12, Vitamin D, and Vitamin E.

Quick tip

Deficiencies in Folic Acid, B6, B12, Vitamin D, and Vitamin E commonly exist even in patients with a normal diet. A Super B complex vitamin is an excellent recommendation for all people and Vitamin D supplementation is particularly important in people who live in the northern part of the country. Milk is fortified with Vitamin D for this reason.

Vitamin A (Retinol) - fat soluble

- Recommended dose: 3000 IU per day for men and 2333 IU per day for women.
- Promotes night vision, stimulates production and activity of white blood cells and therefore helps the immune system, remodels bones, maintains health of the endothelial system (lining of the blood vessels).
- B carotene is a precursor and is generally not toxic. Despite this would still not exceed 25,000 IU per day.
- Sources include liver, fish, dairy, egg yolks, carrots, sweet potatoes, tomatoes, and fortified breakfast cereals
- Excessive amounts may cause nausea, vomiting, liver disease, and birth defects

- Underlying liver disease and alcohol intake increase the risk of hepatotoxicity (liver disease)

Quick tip

Excessive doses of Vitamin A (over 5000 IU per day) may cause severe liver disease!!

B Vitamins- water soluble

- **Thiamine (B1), Riboflavin (B2), Niacin (B3) , Pantothenic acid (B5), Pyridoxine (B6), Biotin, Folic Acid (Folate), and Cobalamin (B12)**
- B vitamins are commonly deficient in a regular diet.
- **Thiamine (B1):** Assists with metabolism of carbohydrates and maintains appropriate nervous system function. Sources include beef, pork, liver, legumes, nuts, and enriched whole grain.
- **Riboflavin (B2):** Assists with processing of protein, carbohydrates, and fats along with maintaining healthy skin. Sources include beef, pork, legumes, eggs, cheese, milk, nuts, and enriched grain.
- **Niacin (B3):** Assists with processing protein and fat along with healthy nervous system, healthy skin, and healthy digestive track. Sources include liver, turkey, tuna, salmon, swordfish, peanuts, beans, cereals, and enriched grains.
- **Pantothenic acid (B5):** Helps process nutrients and production of RBC (red blood cells). Sources include pork, beef, eggs, peanuts, chicken, peas, beans, lentil, lobster, broccoli, and milk.
- **Biotin:** Helps CNS function and absorption of nutrients. Sources include liver, egg yolks, beans, nuts, and tomatoes.
- **Folic Acid:** Recommended dose is 400 mcg per day. Deficiency can result in birth defects such as spina bifida and anencephaly. May decrease heart disease by helping to recycle homocysteine to methionin,

and may lower risk of colon cancer and breast cancer. Sources include green vegetables, dry beans, peas, oranges, and fortified grain.

- **Pyridoxine (B6):** Recommended dose 1.3-1.7 mg per day. May decrease heart disease by helping to recycle homocystein, helps process protein and fat, maintain nervous and immune systems, maintains normal glucose, may help in attention deficit, and may help in premenstrual syndrome. Sources include pork, beef, poultry, fish, eggs, peanuts, bananas, carrots.
- **Cobalamin (B12):** Recommended dose 6 mg per day. Pernicious anemia is an autoimmune related deficiency. Deficiency may result in memory loss, peripheral neuropathy, hallucinations, disorientation, dementia/sources include broccoli, green peppers, spinach, citrus fruits, tomatoes, cabbage, strawberries, and potatoes.

Quick tip

Take a Super B complex daily. Careful with Folic Acid supplements without insuring appropriate Vitamin B12 levels. Folic acid may hide the early signs of B12 deficiency.

Vitamin C (Ascorbic Acid) - water soluble

- Recommended dose: 90 mg per day for men, 75 mg per day for women. Add 35 mg per day for smokers.
- Excellent antioxidant properties.
- Helps control infection, helps make collagen including bones, teeth, gums, blood vessels.
- Sources include citrus, berries, green and red peppers, tomatoes, broccoli, and spinach.
- Deficiency may result in Scurvy.

Vitamin D (Calciferol) - fat soluble

- Recommended dose: up to 50 years old 5 mcg, 51-70 years old 10 mcg, greater than 70 years old 15 mcg. New studies suggest that 25mcg per day (1000 IU) is a better recommendation.
- Exposure to sun helps your skin make Vitamin D. African Americans have a higher incidence of Vitamin D deficiency.
- If you live north of a line stretching from San Francisco to Philadelphia there is a high probability you are deficient due to less total sun exposure time.
- Vitamin D insures adequate absorption of calcium and phosphate which promotes bone formation.
- Deficiency in Vitamin D results in increased fractures. May also increase risk of colon cancer, breast cancer, and prostate cancer.
- Excessive amounts may cause nausea, vomiting, constipation, weight loss, confusion, cardiac arrhythmias.
- Hard to find in foods: Found in fortified milk and cereal along with salmon and tuna.

Vitamin E (Tocopherol) - fat soluble

- Recommended dose: 20-30 IU per day from food.
- Some studies suggest that 400 IU per day may be needed.
- Excellent antioxidant properties which may decrease cancer risk. Probably does not protect against heart disease like originally thought.
- Sources include fish, milk, egg yolks, nuts, fruits, peas, beans, broccoli, spinach, and fortified cereals.
- Excessive doses have very low risk.
- Vitamin E supplementation may "thin" the blood and increase bleeding risk.

Quick tip

Discontinue Vitamin E before surgery as it will increase the intra-operative and post operative bleeding risk. Make sure your physician/surgeon/anesthesiologist is aware of the supplements you are taking.

Vitamin K (Phylloquinone) - fat soluble

- Recommended dose: 80 mcg per day for males, 65 mcg per day for females.
- Helps manufacture 6 of 13 proteins needed for blood clotting.
- Helps with bone formation.
- Sources include green leafy vegetables, broccoli, cabbage, tomatoes, Brussels sprouts, cheese, and cooking oils.

Minerals

Minerals originate from earth and water sources. They are extremely important in multiple metabolic functions ranging from heart, thyroid and immune function to bone and teeth formation.

Calcium

- Promotes bone and teeth formation, assists with blood clotting and muscle/nerve function.
- Sources include salmon, milk, cheese, yogurt, cabbage, and broccoli.
- Excessive doses can result in calcium skin deposits, kidney stones, and decreased magnesium/zinc/iron absorption.

Quick tip

Vitamin D promotes calcium absorption. High phosphate levels interfere with calcium absorption.

Iodine

- Important in thyroid hormone formation.
- Sources include iodized salt, seafood, and kelp.
- Excessive doses can promote thyroid problems. This is more common in people with underlying multi-nodular goiter or autoimmune thyroid disease.
- Deficiency results in a Goiter (enlarged thyroid gland).

Iron

- Supports immune function and red blood cell formation.
- Sources include meat, fish, poultry, lentils, fortified breads and cereal.
- Excessive doses may result in constipation, diarrhea, liver disease, and decreased absorption of zinc/calcium/copper.

Quick tip

Iron overdose may cause liver failure, particularly in children.

Magnesium

- Maintains normal muscle and nerve function, helps with regular heart rhythm, improves bone strength, and improves energy production.
- Sources include meats, seafood, milk, cheese, yogurt, green vegetables, bran cereal, and nuts.
- Excessive amounts may result in diarrhea, muscle weakness, irregular heart rate, kidney failure, and mental status changes.

Phosphorus

- Helps maintain healthy bones and energy.
- Sources include milk, cheese, yogurt, peas, meat, fish, and eggs.
- Excessive doses result in decrease calcium absorption and bone damage.

Zinc

- Supports immune system and promotes wound healing, assists with digestion, and promotes intestinal health.
- Sources include red meat, liver, oysters, milk, some seafood, eggs, beans, and nuts, and whole grain fortified cereal.
- Excessive doses cause decreased iron and copper absorption, decreased HDL, and decreased immune function.

Quick tip

Best daily recommendations:

1. Multiple Vitamin with Minerals once a day
2. Super B Complex once a day
3. Zinc: 25 mg once a day during flu symptoms
4. Calcium: 1500 mg plus Vitamin D daily if living in northern climates, post menopausal women, and patients on chronic steroids

Glycemic Index, Glycemic Load, and My Pyramid

Glycemic Index:

The foundation of the glycemic index (GI) is that not all carbohydrates are created equally. Certain carbs will increase the blood glucose level quickly and therefore create a rapid rise in the insulin level. This will drive the glucose into cells in the body where the glucose may be converted into fat. The lower the glycemic index the slower and longer the glucose rises and therefore will result in less stimulation of insulin production. The lower the glycemic index the better the carbohydrate. The glycemic index of each carb is calculated by studying the glucose response to specific food intake in healthy volunteers. It varies from 0 to 100 (pure glucose).

- **Low Glycemic Index: less than 55**
- **Medium Glycemic Index: 56-69**
- **High Glycemic Index: 70 or more**

Quick Glycemic Index tips:

1. Fructose has a lower GI (19) than sugar (glucose/sucrose- 100)
2. High fructose corn syrup is a misnomer as it contains 50% glucose
3. Use grain products that are either whole wheat, sourdough, rye, pumpernickel, oats, barley, or bran as these will have a lower GI
4. Decrease white potato intake
5. Eat fruits and vegetables. Fruits are better earlier in the day with vegetables any time but particularly in the evening
6. Change to whole wheat pasta and noodles
7. Rice should be brown, wild, or Basmati.
8. Quinoa is an excellent carbohydrate with a lower GI and higher protein content
9. Use high GI carbohydrates when carbohydrate loading or after exercising/athletic competition as the muscles need to replace their glycogen stores

10. Salads with Vinaigrette dressing are the best as the monounsaturated fat in the dressing is healthy and will also delay stomach emptying and lower the GI of the salad

Low Glycemic Index foods- short list:

Cereals:

- Special K - 54
- Oatmeal – 49

Pastas:

- Whole wheat – 43
- Egg Fettuccini – 32

Breads:

- Whole wheat – 49
- Pumpernickel – 50

Vegetables/Legumes:

- Asparagus, Broccoli, Cauliflower, Celery, Cucumber, Green beans, Lettuce, Peppers, Snow peas, Spinach, Squash, Tomatoes, Zucchini – 15
- Beans (various) – 29 to 52

Fruit:

- Grapefruit – 25
- Apples, Pears – 38
- Oranges – 44
- Grapes – 46
- Bananas – 54

Quick tip

Watermelon has a high GI but a low Glycemic load due to the low total carbs per gram of watermelon.

Nuts:

- Peanuts – 13
- Walnuts – 15
- Cashews – 25

Juice:

- Apple juice – 41
- Pineapple juice – 46
- Grapefruit juice – 48
- Orange juice – 52

Medium or High Glycemic Index foods- short list:

Grains:

- Brown rice – 55
- White rice – 58

Fruit:

- Raisins – 64
- Pineapple – 66
- Watermelon – 72

Cereals:

- Shredded wheat – 69
- Rice Krispies – 82
- Cornflakes – 83

Breads:

- Cheese pizza – 60
- Hamburger bun – 61

- White bread – 71
- White Bagel - 72
- White rolls – 73

Vegetables:

- French fries – 75
- Mashed potatoes – 80

Glycemic Load

The Glycemic Load (GL) factors in the actual amount of carbohydrates in each product. The calculation is: GI divided by 100 X net carbs. A food that has a low amount of carbs per gram of weight will have less effect on the blood glucose level. A classic example is watermelon which has a high GI but is actually mostly water and therefore the amount of carb intake per serving is fairly low making the total carb intake low.

- **Low GL: 10 or less**
- **Medium GL: 11-19**
- **High GL: greater than 20**

My Pyramid

This is the US Government (USDA) recommendations on healthy eating habits. It is a well thought out guideline which breaks the food groups into five categories:

My Pyramid breakdown:

- **Grains:** (Orange stripe on the pyramid): 1 oz is one slice of bread or 1 cup of breakfast cereal or ½ cup of cooked rice/cereal/pasta. Eat 6 oz daily with an emphasis on whole wheat products.

- **Vegetables:** (Green stripe): 2 ½ cups daily with varied intake from dark green to orange to beans and peas.
- **Fruits:** (Red stripe): 2 cups daily. Eat a variety of fresh, frozen, canned, or dried fruit. Careful with canned fruit and only use the fruit canned in its own juice. Also be careful with dried fruits due to the high fructose corn syrup (HFCS) content. Go easy on the fruit juices and make sure the product is truly fruit juice.
- **Milk:** (Blue stripe): 3 cups per day. Stick with the low fat or fat free products when choosing milk, yogurt, or other milk products. If you are lactose intolerance select the lactose free varieties or take Lactaid tablets before eating. If this fails choose other high calcium foods or take calcium with Vitamin D supplement.
- **Meat and Beans:** (Purple stripe): 5 ½ oz daily. Select low fat or lean meats and poultry. Vary your protein routine with meats, poultry, fish, legumes (beans and peas), nuts, and seeds.
- **Oils:** (Yellow stripe): Very small component of the daily intake. Try to obtain your oil from fish (salmon, etc), nuts, and liquid oils such as olive oil and canola oil (high in Omega-3) or corn oil and soybean oil (high in Omega-6). Pay attention to the Omega-3 intake as generally this requires supplemention.

Pyramid tips:

- At least ½ of your grain intake should be whole grain. (higher per my recommendation).
- Vary your veggies. Consume dark green, orange, etc. (Red, yellow, etc also excellent per my recommendations).
- Focus on fruits. Eat them for meals, snacks, etc. Careful with fruit juice intake. (Real fruit juice such as orange or apple is OK in moderation). Generally concentrate on fruit intake in the first 2/3 of the day and also use fruits in a dessert situation. (All per my recommendations).
- Get your calcium rich food. Particularly low fat or fat free dairy products.
- Go lean with protein. Low fat chicken or turkey (white meat is lower in fat), low fat meat (top sirloin, low fat hamburger), and fish. Add in legumes such as beans and peas for protein.

- Change your oil. Get oil from fish, nuts, and liquid oils such as Olive oil, Canola oil, Corn oil, and Soybean oil. Olive oil is clearly the single best choice.
- Don't sugarcoat it. Avoid foods that have sugar and sweeteners as their first ingredient.
- Establish an exercise routine.
- Limit TV and Computer time.
- Give gifts that encourage exercise.

Body Fat and Body Mass Index (BMI)

The BMI and Body fat measurements assist in providing an objective, reproducible method of diagnosing obesity. Despite this goal, there are significant deficiencies with most methods currently employed. The Body Mass Index (BMI) is the widely used as it is easy to calculate with simple measurements but the Body Fat measurements are the most accurate particularly with the Dexa, Underwater weighing, and Air out methods. Any method employed should be used in combination with a physician's clinical evaluation of the individual's body type.

Body Mass Index

BMI is a calculation that provides an indication of the level of obesity in a given individual. Insurance companies will look at the BMI to assist in determining the insurability of an individual. The major problem with the BMI is that muscle weighs more than fat and a muscular, athletic type body will have a high BMI even when they are not clinically obese. Many well known professional athletes have a high BMI and would be considered obese based on this calculation. In reality there body fat is low and they are truly in excellent physical condition. The interpretation of the BMI should include a description of the body type.

- **BMI Calculation:** Weight in pounds X 703/ height in inches/ height in inches. There are many web sites which allow you to put in the appropriate numbers and the BMI will be calculated for you.
- **BMI Interpretation:**
    1. Underweight: less than 18.5
    2. Healthy: 18.5-24.9
    3. Overweight: 25-30
    4. Obese: 30-40
    5. Extremely Obese: greater than 40

Body Fat

Measurement of the percentage of body fat provides a more accurate indication of obesity. The measurement must be done with a reproducible method.

- **Skinfold calipers:** Use small pinching calipers and measure the skin folds in 3-9 places. This method requires training and in untrained hands the results can vary by as much as 6%. Acceptable as a rough screening method but overall unreliable. Best is to measure multiple sites using the Parillo method. This requires multiple measurement sites which increase the accuracy. Measurements are made in the chest, abdominal, suprailiac, bicep, tricep, thigh, subscapular, lower back, and calf. Each measurement in millimeters is made from the right side of the body and each measurement is done twice to insure accuracy. If the two measurements vary by more than 1-2mm, then redo the measurements. To calculate the body fat enter the measurements either in your own computer program or on line. An excellent web site is Body Tracker.
- **Bioelectrical impedance:** Step on a scale or hold on to hand grips and a small electrical current is sent through the body. Fat blocks the signal more than muscle and this creates the measurement. Overall this method is not particularly accurate.
- **Underwater weighing:** This method works on the premise that fat floats and muscle sinks. The person sits in a tank of water, blows out their air, and goes underwater. They then sit on an underwater weight scale. This method is quite accurate and reproducible.
- **Air out:** Another accurate method is the use of a BOD POD. This is a fiberglass egg shaped chamber where the person is encased in the chamber and computer sensors measure how much air your body displaces. This method is equally accurate to the underwater weighing.
- **DEXA (Dual Energy X Ray Absorptiometry):** This method uses a dose of 2 different X ray energies that can measure the fat content in a body. It is very accurate overall but expensive. Dexa uses the equipment that was developed to measure bone density.

Normal Body Fat

- **Men:** 12-20%
- **Women:** 16-26%. Higher for women due to the reproductive fat (hips, thighs, etc.)

Quick tip

BMI is a commonly used method for determining obesity, but remember people with a higher muscle mass will have a higher BMI even when they are not clinically obese.

Meat/Poultry/Pork/Fish/Shellfish Nutritional Information

Meat:

Optimum is Top Sirloin and trim off the fat. Filet is a closed second choice.

Excellent source for:

- Protein (high quality)
- Iron
- Calcium
- B12
- Zinc
- B6
- Selenium
- Phosphorus
- Riboflavin

Poultry:

Optimum is white meat chicken or turkey.

Excellent source for:

- Protein
- Calcium
- Magnesium
- Phosphorus
- Potassium
- Selenium
- Niacin
- B6
- Vitamin A

Pork:

Optimum is pork loin and trim off the fat.

Excellent source for:

- Protein (high quality)
- Iron
- Magnesium
- Phosphorus
- Potassium
- Zinc
- Thiamine
- Riboflavin
- B12
- B6

Fish:

Optimal choice is Orange roughy or Salmon.

Excellent source for:

- Protein (high quality)
- Omega-3 (cold water fish)
- B6
- B12
- Vitamin A and D (particularly oily fish)
- Calcium (lower amounts)
- Phosphorus
- Magnesium
- Potassium

Quick tip

Careful with excess mercury in certain fish particularly swordfish, shark, king mackerel, and tilefish.

Scallops:

Excellent source for:

- Protein
- B12
- Omega-3
- Phosphorus
- Magnesium
- Potassium
- Vitamin A
- Folate
- Tryptophan

Shrimp:

Excellent source for:

- Protein
- Omega-3
- Selenium
- B12
- Vitamin D
- Niacin
- Minerals- Zinc, Copper, Magnesium
- Tryptophan
- Iron

Animal/Fish protein source breakdown

—

Food type	Calories	Total fat (gms)	Saturated fat (gms)	Cholesterol (mg)
Chicken (3oz)				
Breast- no skin	140	3.1	0.9	73
Leg- no skin	162	7.1	2.0	80
Thigh- no skin	178	9.3	2.6	81
Turkey (3oz)				
Breast- no skin	161	4	0.5	80
Pork (3oz)				
Tenderloin	120	3.0	1.0	62
Top loin chop	173	5.2	1.8	61
Center loin chop	153	6.2	1.8	72
Beef (3oz)				
Top sirloin	162	7.1	2.2	76
Tenderloin	175	8.1	3.0	71
Eye of Round	141	4.0	1.5	59
Fish (3oz)				
Orange roughy	75	0.8	0.0	22
Tilapia	96	1.7	0.6	50
Cod	89	0.7	0.1	40
Flounder	99	1.3	0.3	58
Halibut	119	2.5	0.4	35
Salmon	175	11.0	2.1	54
Shellfish (3oz)				
Shrimp	84	0.9	0.2	166
Scallops	113	3.4	0.6	34

Quick tip

Best options in each category are Chicken breast, Turkey breast, Top sirloin, Pork tenderloin, Orange Roughy, and Salmon (for cold water fish and high Omega-3). Remember that dairy, legumes (beans), eggs, and nuts are all excellent sources of protein. Eggs protein is considered the ultimate protein. All of the protein in eggs are found in the egg white.

Fruit Nutritional Details

Apples

- Low calorie (80 Kcal) but higher in carbs (21 grams)
- No sodium, fat, or cholesterol
- High fiber
- Contains Boron which helps bone growth
- Contains phytochemicals
- Apple types
    1. **Red Delicious**: Sweet and juicy.
    2. **Golden Delicious**: Sweet and mellow.
    3. **Fuji**: Sweet, crisp, and juicy.
    4. **Granny Smith**: Tart.
    5. **McIntosh**: Tart and tangy.

Bananas

- Low calorie (80-110Kcal) but higher in carbs (17-29grams)
- No sodium, fat, or cholesterol
- Excellent Vitamin C, Potassium, B6
- High fiber
- Banana types
    1. **Cavendish**: "Normal" banana in the US.
    2. **Manzano**: Smaller but slightly sweeter and drier.
    3. **Nino**: Very small and very sweet- finger banana.
    4. **Red**: Smaller, sweeter, and firmer.

Quick tip

Nino bananas are excellent sweet nutritional snacks. Children in particular love the size and taste.

Berries

- Low calorie (30Kcal) and low carbs (7grams)
- High fiber
- Excellent Phytochemicals and Antioxidants
- Berry types
  1. **Blackberries**: Sweet and juicy.
  2. **Blueberries**: Sweet and juicy.
  3. **Cranberries**: Tart and firm.
  4. **Raspberries**: Includes red, black, and golden- intense flavor but fragile.
  5. **Strawberries**: Smaller are usually sweeter.

Citrus

- Low to medium calorie (15 to 80Kcal)
- Variable carbs (3-21grams)
- Excellent Folate, Potassium, B6, Thiamine, Niacin
- Fantastic Vitamin C content
- High in Phytochemicals and Antioxidants
- No sodium and no fat
- Acceptable fiber content
- Citrus types
  1. **Grapefruit**: 21grams carbs.
  2. **Kumquat**: Minimal carbs, eat unpeeled as rind is sweet, looks like a small orange, inside dry and tart.
  3. **Lemon**: Minimal carbs, use the juice.
  4. **Lime**: Tart and sour, aromatic.
  5. **Key Lime**: Tangy and tart.
  6. **Orange**: Navel excellent eating, Valencia excellent eating and juicing, Temple which is a cross between a tangerine and an orange is excellent for eating.
  7. **Tangerine, Mandarin, Clementine**: Easy to peel and very sweet.

Grapes

- Actually a berry
- May be black, red, or white (green) and may be seedless or with seeds
- Low calorie (60Kcal) but moderate carbs (13-15grams)
- No sodium, no fat, no cholesterol
- Excellent phytochemicals
- Seedless type
    1. **Thompson light green**: Crunchy, sweet, and juicy.
    2. **Red flame seedless**: Crunchy, sweet, and juicy.
    3. **Perletter**: Mild, sweet, and slightly tart.
    4. **Champagne**: Very sweet, wine like.
- White/Green Seeded
    1. **Calmeria**: Mild, sweet, and tangy.
    2. **Museat**: Juicy, intense sweetness, and rich perfume.

Melons

- Low calorie (25-30Kcal) and low carbs (5-8grams)
- No fat or cholesterol
- Minimal sodium
- Excellent Vitamin C and Vitamin A
- Excellent phytochemicals
- Melon types
    1. **Cantaloupe**: Juicy and sweet.
    2. **Honeydew**: Tender and sweet, mixes well with other fruits.
    3. **Crenshaw**: Very sweet.
    4. **Casaba**: Very sweet and juicy.
    5. **Watermelon**: Sweet flavor.

Quick tip

Fresh fruit are excellent snacks with many that are easy to transport and do not require refrigeration. They also may help satisfy a sweet tooth.

Pears

- Low to medium calorie (70-100Kcal)
- Medium carbs (13-26grams)
- No sodium, no fat, no cholesterol
- Excellent Fiber, Vitamins, Minerals
- Excellent antioxidants and phytochemicals
- Pear types
    1. **Bartlett**: Yellow (more ripe) and green- both are succulent and sweet.
    2. **Anjou**: Can be green or red and do not change color- sweet and juicy.
    3. **Comice**: Green with red blush- very sweet juice.
    4. **Seckel**: Maroon and olive skin and do not change color- tiny and ultrasweet.

Stone Fruit- summer fruits

- **Apricots**: Low calorie (15Kcal), low carbs, no sodium, no fat, excellent B carotene, Vitamin C, potassium, and fiber.

- **Cherries:** Low calorie (45Kcal), medium carbs (12grams), no sodium, no fat, excellent B vitamins, Vitamin C, and phytochemicals with a sweet and juicy flavor.
- **Peach:** Low calorie (45Kcal), low carbs, no sodium, no fat, excellent Vitamin A and C, Beta carotene, phytochemicals with a sweet taste.
- **Prunes:** Medium calories (110Kcal), medium carbs, minimal sodium, no fat, excellent potassium, Vitamin A, magnesium, iron, fiber, and antioxidants.
- **Plums:** Low calorie (40Kcal), minimal carbs (10grams), minimal fat (0.5grams), no sodium, excellent Vitamin A and C, and phytochemicals.

Quick tip

Remember, as general rule of thumb for the best carb control, concentrate your fruits earlier in the day with the vegetables any time during the day but particularly later in the day.

Tropical Fruits

- **Star fruit:** (Asia) Excellent Vitamin A, fiber, potassium, and polyphenols (antioxidant for the heart).
- **Papaya:** Excellent fiber, potassium, folate, Vitamin A, and papain.
- **Guava:** (South America) Excellent Vitamin C, carotenoids, and fiber.
- **Passion Fruit:** (South America) Excellent fiber, Vitamin A, and potassium.
- **Uniq Fruit:** (Jamaica) Excellent Vitamin C and carotenoids.

- **Acai**: (Central and South America) Excellent B Vitamins, iron, fiber, omega 9, fatty acids, protein, and antioxidants.
- **Coconut**: High in fat!!! With very high saturated fats.
- **Mango**: Green changes to yellow when ripe with excellent Vitamin A, C, and D. Juicy and sweet, but tart.

Other Fruits

- **Avocado**: Higher calorie and higher fat but excellent "good" fats (unsaturated). Excellent folate, potassium, Vitamin C and E, fiber, and phytochemicals.
- **Date**: Higher carb and higher calorie but no fat and no sodium. Excellent fiber, potassium, B Vitamins, magnesium, and iron.
- **Pineapple**: Excellent Vitamin C, fiber, folate, iron, thiamine, magnesium, and B6.

Quick tip

Avocados are excellent nutritionally despite the higher calorie and higher fat content. The fat is primarily monounsaturated fat which is a "good" fat. Fats are essential for satiety (feeling full) during a meal which prevents overeating.

Vegetable Nutritional Details

Legumes

- This category includes **beans and peas**. They are the edible seeds of pods.
- Overall legumes have excellent protein, folate, potassium, and fiber.
- Low calorie (15-90Kcal) with minimal to no fat:
    1. **Black eyes peas**
    2. **Green peas**
    3. **Lima beans**
    4. **Fava beans**
    5. **Snow peas**
    6. **Green beans**
    7. **Sugar snap peas**
    8. **Yellow wax**
    9. **Chinese long**
- Moderate calories (310-330Kcal) with minimal fat:
    1. **Black beans**
    2. **Pinto beans**
    3. **Red beans**
    4. **French green beans**
    5. **Cranberry beans**
- Moderate calories (190-360Kcal) with moderate fat:
    1. **Garbanzo beans**
    2. **Soybeans- Edamame** (but unsaturated "good" fats)

Cabbages

- Low calorie (15-30Kcal), minimal carbs.
- Low sodium, no fat.
- Cabbage has excellent fiber, folate, calcium, iron, Vitamin K, potassium, Vitamin C, and phytochemicals.
- **Cabbage types:**
    1. **Green**
    2. **Red**

3. Savoy
4. Napa

Quick tip

Cabbage is commonly deficient in American diets, but is a fantastic source of nutrition!! Consider adding this to salads and wraps.

Cucumbers

- Botanically is a fruit but used as a vegetable.
- Low calorie (15-40Kcal) with minimal carbs.
- No sodium, no fat, no cholesterol.
- Cucumbers are an excellent source of Vitamin A, Vitamin C, and potassium.
- **Cucumber types:**
    1. **Common**
    2. **English**
    3. **Japanese**
    4. **Kirby**
    5. **Armenian**

Egg Plants

- Botanically is a fruit but used as a vegetable.
- Low calorie (10Kcal) and low carbs.
- No sodium, no fat.
- Egg plants are an excellent source of fiber and potassium.
- **Egg Plant types:**
    1. **Italian**
    2. **Chinese**

3. **Purple**
4. **White**
5. **Japanese** (higher in carbohydrate content)

Greens

- Low calorie (10-35Kcal) and low carb.
- Minimal sodium, no fat, no cholesterol.
- Greens are an excellent source of Vitamin A/C/E, Beta carotene, calcium, iron, fiber, and potassium.
- **Green Types:**
    1. **Arugula**
    2. **Spinach**
    3. **Endive**
    4. **Collard Greens**
    5. **Kale**
    6. **Turnip Greens**
    7. **Mustard Greens**
    8. **Watercress**

Lettuces

- Low calorie (5-10Kcal), low carb.
- Minimal sodium, no fat, no cholesterol.
- Lettuces are an excellent source of Vitamin A/C, calcium, and iron.
- **Lettuce types:**
    1. **Bibb**
    2. **Boston- Butter**
    3. **Green leaf**
    4. **Iceberg**
    5. **Red leaf**
    6. **Romaine**

Quick tip

The darker green lettuce is the best nutritionally. Iceberg lettuce has a lower nutritional value but does have antioxidants. Add other vegetables and legumes to the salad and increase the nutritional value significantly.

Mushrooms

- Variable calories.
- No sodium, no fat, no cholesterol.
- Mushrooms are excellent sources of B Vitamins, selenium, potassium, and copper.
- Low calorie types (5-25Kcal):
    1. **Baby Portobello**
    2. **Portobello**
    3. **Shitake**
    4. **Enoki**
    5. **Maitake**
- Medium calorie (130-140Kcal):
    1. **Chanterelle**
    2. **Morel**
    3. **Porcini**

Onions

- Low calories (5-50Kcal) with minimal carbs.
- Onions are excellent sources of Vitamin C, potassium, folate, iron, and antioxidants.
- Two types with dry/storage and green/fresh
- **Dry/Storage:**
    1. **Sweet/Spring**
    2. **Red/Italian**

3. **Shallot** (extremely flavorful and is the chefs secret onion flavor, but $$$)
4. **Spanish**
5. **Pearl**
6. **Boiling**
- **Green:**
    1. **Scallions**
    2. **Leek**
    3. **Knob**

Chile Peppers

- Low calorie (0-50Kcal) with low carb.
- No fat and no cholesterol.
- Chile peppers are excellent sources of Vitamin A, Vitamin C, Vitamin E, potassium, and folate.
- Hot and spicy overall but add excellent flavor to a dish.
- **Chile pepper types:**
    1. **Anaheim**
    2. **Cherry** (one of my favorites- add as a side item on a salad)
    3. **Fresno**
    4. **Habanero**
    5. **Jalapeno-Chipotle** (excellent for salsa which can be used as a topping for extra flavor)
    6. **Chilaca**
    7. **Serrano**
    8. **Thai**
    9. **Scotch bonnett**

Sweet Peppers

- Low calorie (10-30Kcal) and low carb.
- No sodium, no fat, no cholesterol.
- Sweet peppers are excellent sources of Vitamin A, B Vitamins, Vitamin C, calcium, and iron.
- Crunchy, mild, and sweet.

- **Sweet Pepper types:**
    1. **Bell- Green/Yellow/Red**
    2. **Cubanelle**
    3. **Sweet Banana**

Quick tip

Vegetables are generally low calorie, low carb, and no fat. What could be a better nutritional source? Add vegetables to the main dish to optimize the taste and nutritional value.

Potatoes- with skin

- Low calorie (50-90Kcal) with moderate carbs (12-13grams).
- No fat and no cholesterol.
- Potatoes are excellent sources of Vitamin C, fiber, potassium, B6, and minerals.
- **Potato types:**
    1. **White**
    2. **Russet**- white and Russet highest carbs
    3. **Yukon Gold**- medium carbs
    4. **Red**- lowest carbs of all potatoes
- **Sweet potatoes and Yams** are not truly potatoes. Yams are higher in carbs and sweet potatoes are an excellent source of Vitamin A.

Quick tip

The potato skin contains the majority of the vitamins and minerals whereas the fluffy part contains the carbohydrate component. To maximize the nutritional value of potatoes you must eat the skin. Red potatoes have the lowest carb level.

Radishes

- Low calories (5-15Kcal) with minimal carbs.
- No sodium, no fat, no cholesterol.
- Radishes are an excellent source of Vitamin C, folate, calcium, potassium, and fiber.
- **Radish types:**
  1. **Red**
  2. **Black**
  3. **White**

Winter Squash

- Low calorie (15-70Kcal) with minimal carbs.
- No sodium, no fat, no cholesterol.
- Winter squash is an excellent source of Vitamin A, Vitamin C, fiber, Beta carotene, riboflavin, and iron.
- **Winter squash types:**
  1. **Acorn**
  2. **Buttercup**
  3. **Butternut**
  4. **Chayote**
  5. **Pumpkin Golden Nugget**
  6. **Kabocha**
  7. **Pumpkin**

Summer Squash

- Low calorie (10-20Kcal) with minimal carbs.
- No sodium, no fat, no cholesterol.

- Summer squash is an excellent source of Vitamin A, Vitamin C, and potassium.
- **Summer Squash types:**
    1. **Spaghetti**
    2. **Yellow**
    3. **Zucchini**

Tomato

- Botanically a fruit but used as a vegetable.
- Low calorie (15-25Kcal) with minimal carbs.
- No sodium, no fat, no cholesterol.
- Tomatoes are an excellent source of antioxidants, phytochemicals, potassium, Vitamin A, Vitamin C, and iron.
- **Tomato types:**
    1. **Beefsteak**
    2. **Cherry**
    3. **Grape**
    4. **Roma**
    5. **Teardrop**

Quick tip

Broccoli and Tomatoes are clearly the best of the best vegetables with Asparagus and Spinach also on the list.

Other Vegetables

- **Asparagus:** Low calorie (15Kcal) with minimal carbs, no fat, no cholesterol, and minimal sodium. Excellent source of Vitamin A, B6, folate, iron, calcium, and phytochemicals.
- **Alfalfa sprouts:** Low calorie (5Kcal) with minimal carbs, no fat, no cholesterol, and no sodium.
- **Artichoke:** Low calorie (60Kcal) with minimal sodium, no fat, and no cholesterol. Excellent source of protein, Vitamin A, Vitamin C, calcium, iron, folate, magnesium, and fiber.
- **Broccoli:** Low calorie (10Kcal), with minimal carbs, no fat, and no cholesterol. Excellent source of potassium, Vitamin A, Vitamin C, riboflavin, calcium, iron, antioxidants, and phytochemicals.
- **Broccoli sprouts:** Low calorie (20Kcal) with minimal carbs, no fat, no cholesterol, and minimal sodium. Excellent source of potassium, Vitamin A, Vitamin C, calcium, iron, phytochemicals, and antioxidants.
- **Brussels sprouts:** Low calorie (20Kcal) with minimal carbs, no fat, no cholesterol, and minimal sodium. Excellent source of Vitamin A/C, fiber, calcium, iron, and phytochemicals.
- **Carrots:** Low calorie (25Kcal) with moderate carbs (6grams), no fat, and no cholesterol. Excellent source of Vitamin A, calcium, and iron.
- **Cauliflower:** Low calorie (10Kcal) with low carbs, no fat, and no cholesterol. Excellent source of Vitamin C, iron, and calcium.
- **Celery:** Low calorie (10Kcal) with minimal carbs, no fat, no cholesterol, and minimal sodium. Celery contains excellent amounts of potassium, Vitamin C, fiber, calcium, and Vitamin A.
- **Corn:** Low calorie (15Kcal) with moderate (17grams) carbs, no fat, and no cholesterol. Excellent source of fiber, Vitamin A, Vitamin C, iron, protein, and potassium.
- **Okra:** Low calorie (15Kcal) with low carbs, no fat, no cholesterol. Excellent source of Vitamin A, Vitamin C, calcium, and iron.

Herbs

- Essentially no calorie, no fat, no cholesterol, no sodium, no to minimal carbs.

- Add herbs to multiple different recipes to increase the flavor and still maintain the nutritional benefit.
- **Fantastic Herbs include:**
    1. **Basil**
    2. **Chives**
    3. **Cilantro**
    4. **Dill**
    5. **Galangeall**
    6. **Garlic**
    7. **Gingerroot**
    8. **Parsley**
    9. **Mint**
    10. **Horseradish**
    11. **Sage**
    12. **Sorrell**
    13. **Thyme**
- **Extra calcium and iron herbs:**
    1. **Bay leaves**
    2. **Tarragon**
    3. **Savory**
    4. **Rosemary**

Quick tip

Herbs are a great way to add taste to any recipe without adding unnecessary calories.

Daily Nutritional Suggestions

A nutritious diet is best achieved with appropriate planning. Set up your meal plans and snacks at least the day before, or even better plan an entire week. Snacks and lunches are particularly important to plan for as these can easily be premade. It is also equally easy to skip a snack when it is not premade. The following are simple, quick suggestions with more extensive options later in the manual.

Quick tips

Vary your selection from day to day as this will prevent boredom in your diet which might result in a trip to McDonalds.

Small servings with each meal or snack are a major key.

Eat the correct foods: Do not obsess with the actual calorie count but remember that we generally underestimate how many calories we consume. Add 25% to your estimated daily caloric intake to obtain a more reasonable guess as to your total daily calories.

Breakfast: The optimum is to start out the morning with home cooking. This will set the nutritional tone for the day.

- Cereal: Kashi, Total, Cheerios, Shredded Wheat, or Special K with or without fresh fruit (sliced banana, berries- raspberries, strawberries, blueberries).
- Oatmeal: Regular or Low sugar Instant (avoid high fructose corn syrup present in many instant brands). Top with sliced bananas or berries or walnuts.
- Eggs/egg beater. Be creative with the additives such as fresh, left over, or frozen vegetables, or top with salsa for extra flavor. Use one egg and then add egg whites for extra protein and to maximize taste. One egg yolk per day is acceptable.
- Center cut Bacon or Turkey bacon.
- Canadian bacon.
- Whole wheat toast or Whole wheat English muffin. Top with a small amount of low fat butter or real fruit low sugar preserves. My personal favorite is a toasted whole wheat English muffin topped with peanut butter and sliced apple. Careful with bagels as they are higher in carbohydrates.
- Smoothie: Combine banana/berries/orange juice/2tbsp vanilla low fat yogurt.
- Fresh Fruit: Fresh banana, citrus, berries, or melon.
- Juicing: Combine apples, berries, pomegranate juice, carrots, and tomatoes. This is a very nutritious and flavorful drink.

Mid Morning Snack

- As per snack list.

Lunch

- Low fat lunchmeat: Turkey or ham with a 3-4oz per serving.
- Tuna fish: 3-4oz made with low fat Miracle Whip or low fat ranch dressing.

- 3-4oz meat serving: Low fat hamburger, chicken, turkey, pork loin, or sirloin: Grilled or baked.
- 3-4oz fish serving: Orange roughy, salmon, or tilapia: Grilled or baked.

Quick tip

Use mustard or low fat Miracle Whip on sandwiches, pitas, or wraps. A distant second choice is low fat Mayo.

- Salad with Romaine lettuce (or other dark green lettuce): Use a low fat vinaigrette based dressing and garnish with fresh vegetables. Add cabbage and/or spinach for even more nutrition.
- Fresh fruit: Grapes, bananas, melons, and citrus are all excellent choices.
- Vegetables: You may consider eating the vegetables separately or add them to a sandwich. Tomatoes, onions, peppers, mushrooms, lettuce, carrots are all excellent considerations.
- Whole wheat bread, whole wheat pita, or whole wheat tortilla are the optimal choices. May also use Sourdough, Pumpernickel, or Rye.
- Low Fat Cottage cheese: 3-4oz. An excellent nutritional addition to cottage cheese is chopped/sliced strawberries, blueberries, raspberries, or sliced pineapple.
- Skim milk: 6-8oz.
- Lettuce wraps: A healthy choice is Boston lettuce or Romaine lettuce rather than Iceberg. Use the lettuce for a sandwich rather than bread or a wrap.

- Frozen meals: Healthy Choice and Lean Cuisine have flavorful healthy options.
- Fluids: Best choices are caffeine free diet soda, green tea, iced tea, crystal light, and water.

Quick tip

Iceberg lettuce has a lower nutritional value compared to other members of the lettuce family.

Mid Afternoon Snack

- As per snack list.

Dinner

- 3-4oz Meat: Top sirloin, low fat hamburger, turkey, chicken, and pork loin are the optimal choices: Grilled or baked.

- 3-4oz Fish: Orange roughy, salmon, tuna, tilapia are all excellent nutritional choices: Grilled or baked.
- 3-4oz Shrimp or Scallops: Grilled or baked.
- Vegetables/Legumes: There are many healthy choices including broccoli, asparagus, tomato, and green beans: Fresh or frozen are equally nutritious: Microwave, steamed, or grilled.
- Small amounts of fruit: Melons, citrus, berries, or grapes. Remember the preference of the fruit carbohydrates earlier in the day with the vegetable carbohydrates any time, but particularly at night.
- Whole wheat pasta with tomato based sauce such as marinara.
- Thin crust pizza (whole wheat is possible) with vegetables and low fat cheese.
- Low fat Cottage cheese. Again consider adding chopped/sliced strawberries, blueberries, raspberries, or sliced pineapple for additional nutrition.
- Skim milk/Nonfat milk: 6-8oz.
- Frozen meals: Healthy choice or Lean Cuisine both have excellent flavorful choices.
- Small amounts of whole wheat bread, sourdough, pumpernickel: Use extra virgin olive oil with pepper and cracked red pepper for dipping or small amounts of low fat butter.
- Fluids: Caffeine free diet soda, green tea, iced tea, crystal light, and water.

Quick tip

Low fat Vinaigrette based dressings are healthier than creamy type salad dressings. My personal favorite is Newman's Low fat Balsamic Vinaigrette Dressing.

Evening snack: Both provide excellent Casein protein which is a long acting protein

- Low fat mozzarella string cheese stick (Sargento brand is my personal favorite).
- Low fat Cottage cheese.

Nutrition quick notes

- Use Monounsaturated or Polyunsaturated fats and be careful with the saturated fats. Best cooking options are the MUFA- Olive oil and Canola oil are the best as they do not break down as easy in high heat. For higher heat use Canola oil.
- No Trans fats as this will rapidly raise the total cholesterol and the LDL (bad component of cholesterol).
- Interesterified fats: These are similar to trans fats but they decrease the HDL (good cholesterol).   Specific names include interesterified soybean oil or stearate rich.
- Careful with High Fructose and High Maltose Corn Syrup as these will cause a rapid release in insulin which drives glucose into the cells where it is converted to fat for storage.
- Do not overeat at one meal or snack. Monitor your serving sizes to prevent. Remember we generally underestimate how much we are eating.
- No regular soda. Caffeine free diet soda is a better choice.
- Careful with processed foods as these are usually high in calories, refined sugar, saturated fat, and sodium.
- Minimal to no alcohol.
- Drink plenty of fluids.
- Maximum coffee 16 oz per day (in some studies up to 24 oz is acceptable).
- Add any seasoning to improve flavor but try to minimize salt and sugar additions.

Snack Options- mid AM and mid PM

Snacks in the mid morning and mid afternoon are the key to maintaining a stable blood insulin level and prevent the rapid serum glucose fluxuations which can drive sugar into the cells where it may be converted into fat. With appropriate small meals and snacks you can take in sufficient calories so you will never be hungry. This will prevent overeating at any one meal.

Quick tip

Prepare snacks the night before and be creative on your combinations. Vary your combinations to prevent boredom.

Fruits

- Clementine orange
- Grapes- seedless the best- red or green
- Apple Slices/whole
- Apple Sauce cup- low sugar
- Light fruit cup- packed in water
- Strawberries/Raspberries/Blueberries
- Banana
- POM: Pomegranate juice
- V8 Fusion

Vegetables: If need be, use a small amount of low fat ranch for dipping purposes

- Celery: with or without peanut butter
- Baby Carrots
- Cauliflower
- Grape Tomatoes

- Broccoli bites
- Artichoke hearts
- Radishes
- Green bean bites
- V8 juice- 4oz
- My favorite: combine celery, baby carrots, and grape tomatoes. Add a small amount of peanut butter to one or two of the celery sticks to help you feel full

Meats

- Turkey Pepperoni
- Beef or Turkey Jerky
- Tuna fish- prepackaged- mix with light Miracle Whip- may also substitute low fat Ranch dressing for the Miracle Whip
- Turkey or Low fat Ham- Healthy Choice or Hormel

Cheese

- Light String Cheese (Sargento)
- Jarlsberg light- excellent taste with a lower fat content
- Low fat Baby Bell- a favorite of mine
- Cabot 50% reduced fat sharp
- Athenos low fat Feta cheese
- Kraft 2% Milk Sharp cheddar
- Laughing Cow low fat Swiss- for spreading on pretzel thins or whole wheat crackers

Dairy/Eggs

- Hard Boiled egg
- Light smoothie- premade (Light and Fit Strawberry Banana) or better yet make your own
- Yogurt- Vanilla low fat (best choice Light and Fit), may add sliced/chopped/whole strawberries/raspberries/blueberries/bananas. For extra crunch add a teaspoon of low fat granola
- Light Cottage Cheese- also very good with sliced/chopped/whole strawberries, raspberries, blueberries, bananas

Nuts and Trail Mix: 1oz serving

- Almonds
- Pistachios
- Walnuts
- Pecans
- Planters Trail Mix: Berry, Nut, and Chocolate

Crunchy snacks

- Pretzels
- Pepperidge Farm Whole Wheat Goldfish Cheddar Crackers
- Pretzel thins: with or without low fat cheese spread (my favorite: Light Laughing Cow Original Swiss- excellent as you can limit your snack to one triangle of cheese)
- Whole wheat crackers- with/without low fat cheese spread
- Low fat Whole Wheat Triskets- with/without low fat cheese spread
- Baked chips/tortillas- add salsa with minimal additional calories
- Newman's Own Low fat Pop Corn, butter flavored
- Sun Chips Original

Snack Bars

- Special K Protein Bar
- Pria Carb Select
- South Beach Snack Bar
- Cascadian Farm Organic
- Kashi TLC
- Fiber One Oats and Chocolate

Cookies (try to avoid but cravings do occur)

- Ginger snaps
- Nilla (Vanilla) Wafers reduced fat
- Teddy Grahams Oatmeal
- Snack Wells crème sandwich

Quick tip

Buy a small soft cooler and use this daily to keep your snack fresh and prevent food related illnesses.

Best Frozen Foods

Healthy frozen foods should be kept in the house for those meals or snacks that require a short preparation time. The major problem with all frozen foods is the amount of sodium used to increase taste. If a frozen dish is used then you should be extra careful on the amount of sodium used for the other meals. Generally a 4 gram per day sodium diet is extremely healthy. They can also be used for snacks when your sweet tooth takes control.

Chicken/Turkey

- Healthy Choice Turkey with mixed vegetables and mashed potatoes
- Healthy Choice Sesame Chicken: 230 calories/4.5 grams total fat/1 gram saturated fat/600 mg sodium
- Lean Cuisine Chicken Teriyaki: 300 calories/3.5 grams total fat/1 gram saturated fat/880 mg sodium
- Lean Cuisine Chicken Marsala: 140 calories/4 grams total fat/1.5 gram saturated fat/620 mg sodium
- Weight Watchers Smart Ones Chicken Parmesan: 290 calories/5 grams total fat/1.5 grams saturated fat/630mg sodium

Beef

- Lean Cuisine Steak Tips Portobello: 180 calories/7 grams total fat/2 grams saturated fat/460 mg sodium
- Lean Cuisine Steak, Cheddar, and Mushroom Panini: 310 calories/4.5 grams total fat/1.5 grams saturated fat/600 mg sodium
- Stouffer's Green Pepper Steak: 240 calories/4 grams total fat/1.5 grams saturated fat/910 mg sodium

Fish

- Healthy Choice Café Steamers Creamy Dill Salmon: 240 calories/6 grams total fat/2.5 grams saturated fat/600 mg sodium
- Gortons Grilled Salmon Lemon Butter: 1 filet/100 calories/3 grams total fat/0.5 grams saturated fat/300 mg sodium (but only the salmon, no side items. Easily add 1 cup mixed frozen vegetables)

Quick tip

Frozen foods use a high sodium content to maintain taste. When having a frozen meal, be sure to be extra careful on the sodium content for the remainder of the meals and snacks on that day. 4 grams of sodium per day is a reasonable goal.

Vegetarian

- Boca Burgers: 1 burger/90 calories/3 grams total fat/1 gram saturated fat/280 mg sodium. Excellent protein content.
- Kashi Black Bean Mango: 340 calories/8 grams total fat/1 gram saturated fat/430 mg sodium
- Stouffers Spinach Mozzarella Pizza: 270 calories/6 grams total fat/1.5 grams saturated fat/500 mg sodium

Pasta

- Healthy Choice Chicken Fettuccini Alfredo: 300 calories/5 grams total fat/2 grams saturated fat/430 mg sodium
- Kashi Chicken Pasta Pomodoro: 280 calories/6 grams total fat/1.5 grams saturated fat/470 mg sodium
- Weight Watcher's Smart Ones Three Cheese Ziti Marinara: 290 calories/7 grams total fat/2.5 grams saturated fat/530 mg sodium

- Birds Eye Voila Pesto Chicken Primavera: 210 calories/7 grams total fat/2 grams saturated fat/590 mg sodium

Pizza

- Lean Cuisine Cheese Pizza
- Healthy Choice Gourmet Supreme Pizza: 360 calories/4 grams total fat/1.5 grams saturated fat/900 mg sodium
- Lean Pockets Deli Style Pepperoni Pizza: 270 calories/7 grams total fat/2.5 grams saturated fat/900 mg sodium

Breakfast Entrees

- South Beach Diet Breakfast Wraps: 190 calories/6 grams total fat/2 grams saturated fat/480 mg sodium
- Eggo Nutri-Grain Whole Wheat Waffles: 1 waffle/90 calories/3 grams total fat/0.75 grams saturated fat/210 mg sodium (add fresh fruit topping or low calorie maple syrup)

Quick tip

My personal favorites include:

1. Healthy Choice Turkey with mixed vegetables and mashed potatoes
2. Lean Cuisine Cheese Pizza
3. Lean Pockets Deli Style Pepperoni Pizza
4. Boca Burger
5. South Beach Breakfast Wraps

Treats

- Popsicle Sugar Free Cherry, Orange, Grape: 15 calories/0 fat/0 sugar
- Klondike Slim-a-Bear 100 calorie Chocolate Sandwich: 100 calorie/1.5 grams total fat/1 gram saturated fat/10 grams sugar
- Fudgsicle Original: 100 calories/2 grams total fat/2 grams saturated fat/14 grams sugar
- Skinny Cow Vanilla with Caramel Low Fat Ice Cream Cone: 150 calories/3 grams total fat/2 grams saturated fat/19 grams sugar

Ice Cream

- Haagen-Dazs Low Fat Chocolate Sorbet: ½ cup/130 calories/.5 gram total fat/0 grams saturated fat/20 grams sugar
- Edy's Slow Churned Rich & Creamy Black Cherry Vanilla Swirl Yogurt: ½ cup/100 calories/3 grams total fat/1.5 grams saturated fat/13 grams sugar
- Ben & Jerry's Berried Treasure Sorbet: ½ cup/110 calories/0 grams total fat/24 grams sugar

Quick tip

Treats and Ice Cream have little nutritional value but are important in blunting your desires for unhealthy desserts.

Healthy Recipes

Breakfast

Cereal

Multigrain Cheerios, Special K, Total, or Kashi are all excellent choices: top with sliced banana, strawberries, raspberries, or blueberries (or a combination). Use Skim/Nonfat Milk.

Beverage: 6 oz Orange Juice or 6 oz Apple Juice.

Oatmeal

Cook regular Oatmeal and top with a small amount of low fat butter and skim milk. Add cantaloupe or honeydew as a side fruit or top the oatmeal with blueberries, raspberries, or strawberries.

Beverage: 6 oz Skim Milk and small cup of black coffee.

Quinoa Oatmeal

Combine one cup cooked quinoa (KEEN-wah) with ½ cup skim milk and one tsp low fat butter. Then microwave for 1 minute. Remove and stir. Top with fresh blueberries, raspberries, or strawberries. To cook the Quinoa, bring to a boil a large pot of water with a pinch of salt. Add quinoa, lower the heat and cook until tender (approximately 20 minutes). Drain the water. The quinoa can be stored in the refrigerator.

Beverage: 6 oz Skim Milk

Egg Beater or Scrambled Eggs

Use scrambled eggs or egg beater with any combination of chopped tomato, onion, mushroom, green onions, green or red peppers. Spray the pan with Pam, then sauté the vegetables, add the eggs, and later top with low fat American or Cheddar cheese. Add ½ whole wheat English muffin with low fat butter.

Beverage: 6 oz Orange Juice or 6oz Apple Juice.

Fried or Poached Egg

Use 1 or 2 eggs and cook to your preference. Add one slice of whole wheat or sourdough toast (or English muffin) with low fat butter. Add a side of Turkey bacon or Canadian bacon if you wish.

Beverage: 6 oz Orange Juice or 6 oz Apple Juice.

Apple/Peanut Butter Whole Wheat or Sourdough Bagel

Toast ½ whole wheat bagel, add a smear of peanut butter, and top with sliced apples.

Beverage: 6 oz Skim Milk with a small cup black coffee.

Egg Tortilla

Whole wheat tortilla or flat bread warmed. Fill with scrambled eggs or egg beater, fat free sour cream, salsa, chopped green onions, low fat cheddar or American cheese, and chopped cilantro. Cook the cilantro with the eggs. May also add chopped turkey bacon or turkey sausage.

Beverage: 6 oz Skim milk.

Quick Fiesta Scramble

Use crumbled Turkey sausage or Soy sausage sautéed in a skillet sprayed with Pam. Scramble two eggs (mix with chopped Cilantro and chopped green onion if you wish) and cook with the sausage. Top with low fat Mexican blend shredded cheese (or low fat shredded cheddar cheese) and salsa, then serve.

Beverage: 6 oz Skim milk.

Spinach and Mushroom Omelet

Scramble 2 eggs with spinach (fresh or frozen), sliced mushrooms, chopped green onions, and low fat feta cheese. Top with sliced avocado and sprinkle with parsley. Add a side of whole wheat English muffin.

Beverage: 6 oz Orange Juice or 6 oz Apple Juice.

Egg English Muffin

Toast one half whole wheat or sourdough English muffin (or whole English muffin if you prefer) top with one fried egg (yolk broken and cooked with the white), one slice low fat American cheese, and high fructose corn syrup free catsup (or low fat butter). Add Center Cut Bacon, Turkey bacon, Canadian bacon, Turkey sausage, or soy sausage if you wish.

Beverage: 6 oz Orange Juice or 6 oz Apple Juice.

Smoothie

Smoothie- see list. Add one half toasted whole wheat or sourdough English muffin with small amount of low fat butter.

Beverage: small cup of black coffee.

Breakfast Bars

Choice of Special K, South Beach, Cereal Bars: There are many excellent choices but be careful with the HFCS content. Experiment so you know your preferences and be sure to vary the flavors to maintain interest.

Beverage: 6 oz Skim milk and small cup black coffee.

Low fat/Healthy Pancakes

For a quick breakfast, reconstitute a low fat pancake mix and cook in a pan or on a griddle. Use Pam to prevent sticking. Top with low fat Maple syrup or with fresh fruit (bananas, strawberries, blueberries, and/or raspberries).

- **Option 1: Applesauce pancakes:** Combine 1 ½ cups whole wheat flour, ¾ cup applesauce, 1 cup nonfat milk, 2 egg whites lightly beaten, 1 tsp baking powder, ½ tsp cinnamon, and ¾ tsp vanilla extract. Directions: Mix flour and baking powder in a bowl then slowly stir in the other ingredients. Spray griddle with Pam and cook.
- **Option 2: Blueberry Oatmeal pancakes:** Combine 1 cup water, ½ cup whole wheat flour, ¾ cup instant oatmeal, ¾ cup nonfat milk, 4 egg whites lightly beaten, 1 cup fresh blueberries, 1 tsp baking powder, and ½ tsp sea salt. Directions: Combine oats and water and cook as directed on instant oats package. In one bowl mix baking powder, flour, and salt. In a second bowl mix milk and eggs. Then mix bowl 1 and 2. Finally stir in the oatmeal and blueberries. Spray griddle with Pam and cook.
- **Topping options:** Low fat Maple syrup, fresh fruit, fresh fruit low fat yogurt, honey, or low-cal jam all work very well. Excellent low-cal jam choices include low-cal Polaner, Bionature organic fruit spread, Smucker's low sugar, or St. Dalfour 100% fruit.

Beverage: 6 oz Orange Juice or 6 oz Apple Juice.

Quick Breakfast

1 slice toasted whole wheat raisin bread topped with 1tbsp of peanut butter. Side of low fat French vanilla yogurt mixed with sliced strawberries, blueberries, or raspberries.

Beverage: 6 oz Skim milk.

Yogurt and Fruit

Low fat French vanilla yogurt mixed with sliced or chopped strawberries, whole or chopped raspberries, sliced bananas, or whole blueberries. Add a scoop of low fat granola for crunch if you wish.

Beverage: 6 oz Orange juice.

Quick tip

Granola does not automatically mean healthy. Choose low fat granola and be sure there is no added high fructose corn syrup (HFCS).

Smoothies

1. **Banana/Mixed Berries**: Blend one banana, 1 cup frozen or fresh mixed berries, 2 tbsp low fat vanilla yogurt, and 4oz orange juice.
2. **Banana/Strawberry**: Blend one banana, 1 cup frozen or fresh strawberries, 2 tbsp low fat vanilla yogurt, 3oz orange juice, and 3oz apple juice.
3. **Banana/Raspberry**: Blend one banana, 1 cup raspberries, 2 tbsp low fat vanilla yogurt, 3oz orange juice, and 3oz apple juice.
4. **Mixed Berry**: Blend 1 ½ cup frozen or fresh mixed berries, 2 tbsp low fat vanilla yogurt, 6oz orange juice.
5. **Strawberry/Apple**: Blend 1 cup frozen or fresh strawberries, one slice apple, 2 tbsp low fat vanilla yogurt, and 6oz orange juice.
6. **Peanut butter/Banana**: Blend 2 tbsp peanut butter, one banana, one cup whey protein, 4oz skim milk, and 4 tbsp chocolate frozen fat free yogurt.
7. **Blueberry/Mango**: Blend one cup frozen or fresh blueberries, one cup frozen or fresh mango, and 6oz pineapple juice.

Lunch

Standard Drinks

Water, Diet caffeine free soda, Iced Tea caffeine free, Crystal light

Quick tip

If you have time consider using the dinner recipes for lunch.

Tuna fish wrap

Prepare water packed tuna fish with chopped sweet or red onion (shallots are also a great onion change), chopped celery, sweet relish, and chopped hard boiled egg. Add black pepper and garlic powder, then mix with low fat Miracle Whip or Fat Free Ranch Dressing. Place in a whole wheat wrap with chopped romaine lettuce and chopped tomato.

> ** May substitute whole wheat bread or sourdough bread or whole wheat pita. Also consider a lettuce wrap (Boston lettuce is the better nutritional choice but iceberg is acceptable. If a lettuce wrap is used then skip the chopped Romaine).
>
> Side: One cup red seedless grapes.

Tuna fish wrap #2

Prepare water packed tuna fish with chopped onion and chopped green olives. Add black pepper, garlic powder, and a splash of lemon juice. Mix with low fat Miracle Whip or Fat Free Ranch Dressing. Place in whole wheat wrap with chopped tomato and chopped romaine lettuce.

> ** May substitute whole wheat bread or sourdough bread or whole wheat pita. Also consider a lettuce wrap (Boston lettuce is the better nutritional choice but iceberg is acceptable. If a lettuce wrap is used then skip the chopped Romaine).

> Side: One cup red seedless grapes.

Turkey wrap or Low fat Ham wrap

Place turkey or low fat ham in a whole wheat wrap (or Boston lettuce wrap) with chopped romaine lettuce (skip with the lettuce wrap), chopped tomato, low fat Jarlsberg cheese. Consider adding chopped onion, chopped cucumber, chopped celery, chopped green or red peppers, and chopped carrots. Sprinkle with black pepper and add low fat Miracle Whip or Mustard.

> Side: Cubed Cantaloupe and Honeydew melon.

Quick tip

Nutritious toppings include low fat Miracle Whip, mustard, vinegar/oil olive, and low fat Ranch dressing. There are many different flavored mustard which can improve the taste of a sandwich or wrap. Also consider using different vinegars such as red wine and balsamic combined with extra virgin olive oil.

Turkey sandwich or Low fat Ham sandwich

Place low fat turkey or low fat ham on one or two slices of whole wheat or sourdough or rye bread. You may also substitute whole wheat Pita bread. Top with romaine lettuce, sliced tomato, sliced onion, sliced cucumber, and low fat Jarlsberg cheese. Sprinkle with black pepper and add low fat Miracle whip or mustard.

Side: 1 cup blueberries and raspberries.

Vegetable/Cheese Wrap

Whole wheat wrap loaded with low fat Jarlsberg cheese, low fat American cheese, chopped romaine lettuce, chopped tomato, chopped onion, chopped cucumber, and chopped mushrooms. Add chopped celery, chopped carrots, and chopped red or green peppers if you wish. Sprinkle with black pepper and add low fat Miracle Whip or mustard or Fat Free Ranch Dressing.

** May substitute Whole Wheat Bread, Sourdough Bread or Whole Wheat Pita and use sliced vegetables. Also consider a lettuce wrap (Boston lettuce is the better nutritional choice but iceberg is acceptable. If a lettuce wrap is used then skip the chopped Romaine).

Side: Sliced bananas and strawberries.

Barbecue Chicken Pita

Mix precooked chicken with 1 tbsp barbecue sauce, then microwave. Place in a whole wheat pita and add chopped romaine lettuce, chopped cucumber, chopped tomato, and Fat Free Ranch Dressing.

Side: Cubed cantaloupe and honeydew melon.

Chicken or Shrimp Tortilla Roll

Use precooked chopped chicken or shrimp and place in a whole wheat tortilla. Add chopped onion, chopped romaine lettuce, and low fat Feta cheese. Roll and grill using Pam to prevent sticking to the pan. Use Salsa for dipping.

Side: Baked Tortilla chips dipped in salsa with one cup of red grapes.

Grilled Cheese with sliced Tomato

Whole wheat bread or Sourdough bread layered with low fat American cheese and sliced tomato. Also consider adding sliced sweet onion if you wish. Use low fat butter on the outside of the bread and grill using Pam to prevent sticking.

Side: Pretzels and banana stuffed with small amount of peanut butter then sliced.

Turkey Reuben

Use two slices of rye bread and butter the outside with low fat butter. Drain canned sauerkraut and mix with low fat thousand island dressing and low fat feta cheese. Spread this on the rye bread and top with low fat turkey (Healthy Choice is excellent) and low fat Jarlsberg cheese (or low fat Swiss cheese). Grill on a pan sprayed with Pam.

Side: Pretzels and a cup of grapes.

Quick lunch

Healthy Choice or Lean Cuisine Frozen dinner: Chicken, Turkey, and Salmon are the best choices.

Side: Clementine or grapes or banana or cantelope/honeydew or blueberries/strawberries.

Bagel delite

Whole wheat bagel with small amount of low fat Miracle whip or mustard. Consider substituting Hummus as a smear. Top with 1 slice red onion, 1 slice beefsteak tomato, leaf Romaine or Boston lettuce, and sliced cucumbers. Add low fat turkey or low fat ham if you wish.

Side: Banana or 1 cup Blueberries/Raspberries.

Quick Pizza

½ Whole wheat English muffin topped with marinara sauce, garlic powder, low fat parmesan cheese, and low fat mozzarella cheese. Top with your choice of Turkey Pepperoni, red or sweet onions, sliced mushroom, and/or green/red peppers for extra taste. For a white pizza use sliced tomatoes (Roma tomatoes are an excellent choice) instead of the marinara sauce.

Side: One cup of Red Grapes.

Lunch Turkey or Ham Kebabs

Cube low fat deli turkey and/or low fat deli ham and cube low fat cheddar cheese. Thread onto a skewer alternating with grapes and dried apricots.

Salsa Recipes

Tomato Salsa

One small can petite diced tomatoes, ½ chopped sweet or red onion, chopped green onion, chopped fresh cilantro, one seeded and chopped jalapeno pepper. Season to taste with black pepper, sea salt, garlic powder, oregano, and basil. Add a splash of lime juice if you wish.

- For extra zip add cayenne pepper and leave the seeds of the jalapeno pepper in the mixture.

Mango Salsa

Skin and remove seeds of a mango and cut in cubes and skin and pit an avocado and cut in cubes. Mix with ½ chopped sweet or red onion, chopped green onion, chopped cilantro, seeded and chopped jalapeno pepper and 1 tbsp lime juice. Then season to taste with garlic powder or minced garlic.

Quick tip

Salsa is a great way to add taste to the meal and still maintain an excellent nutritional value. Combine with baked chips for the optimal appetizer or snack, and use as a topping on meat or fish.

Vegetables/Legumes/Side Salads

Steamed or Microwave Broccoli, Green Beans, Peas, Asparagus, Mixed Vegetables, Brussels sprouts, Zucchini, or Corn

Use Fresh or Frozen vegetables as they are both equally nutritious. Steam or microwave with a covered dish or a steamer zip lock bag. Top with low fat butter or even better use the garlic butter sauce below.

- Garlic Butter Sauce: Melt low fat butter with garlic powder, onion powder, black pepper, and pinch of dried oregano, basil, and sea or kosher salt. Pour over vegetables after cooking, toss or stir, and then drain off the excess before serving.

Sliced Zucchini and Yellow Squash Medley

Steam or microwave the zucchini and yellow squash 3-5 minutes then sprinkle with sea or kosher salt, black pepper, and low fat Parmesan cheese. Toss and serve.

Grilled Asparagus, Zucchini, Red Bell Pepper, Red or Sweet Onion slices, and Portobello mushroom slices

Brush the vegetables with extra virgin olive oil, then sprinkle with black pepper (or pepper blend), garlic powder, oregano, basil, and a pinch of sea or kosher salt. Grill until tender. Be careful not to over grill the vegetables. Asparagus in particular cooks very quickly. Use one or any combination with a meal. The optimum time to use this vegetable prep is when you are grilling your main course. Cleanup becomes a snap.

Mushrooms and Onions with Soy Sauce

Combine sliced mushrooms (any combination) with sliced sweet onions. Sauté the vegetables in extra virgin olive oil then add low sodium soy sauce (Kikoman's is the best). Finally sprinkle with pepper and oregano, toss and serve. Do not add salt due to the low sodium soy sauce.

Roasted Vegetables

Slice lengthwise red bell pepper, zucchini, and yellow squash. Add trimmed Asparagus. Toss the vegetables in a mixture of 4 tsp extra virgin olive oil, 1 tbsp minced garlic, 1 tsp balsamic vinegar, with a pinch of sea or kosher salt, basil, and black pepper. Spread on a baking sheet sprayed with Pam and bake at 450 degrees F for 25-30 minutes.

Corn on the Cob

Place corn ears (white or bi-colored are sweeter) in cold water with a pinch of salt, and then bring water to a boil. Roll in low fat butter and sprinkle with black pepper. Consider grilling the corn if you are using the grill. The corn can be grilled in or out of the husk.

Baked Potato with Skin

Use a small Russet or Yukon gold potato and cook in the microwave or oven. Split potato open and garnish with fat free sour cream, parsley, and black pepper. Remember the skin contains most of the nutrients in a potato, so eat the skin. Yukon gold potatoes have less starch content.

Vegetable Brown Rice

Sauté in extra virgin olive oil for 2-3 minutes a combination of minced garlic and finely chopped sweet onion. Add chopped red bell pepper and chopped celery, then sauté another 2-3 minutes. Finally add one cup instant brown rice, 1 ½ cups water, and sea or kosher salt. Bring the mixture to a boil, reduce heat, and simmer covered for 5 minutes. Remove from the heat, stir in parsley and black pepper before serving. For a change up sauté the vegetables and then combine with precooked quinoa (KEEN-wah). Stir in the parsley and black pepper and serve.

Quinoa side dish

Microwave broccoli florets and place to the side. Bring to a boil a large pot of water with a pinch of sea salt. Add one cup of quinoa (KEEN-wah), lower the temperature and cook until tender (approximately 20 minutes). Then combine the quinoa and broccoli 2 tbsp of low fat feta cheese, kalamata olives, 4 tbsp chopped sun dried tomatoes, 1 tbsp balsamic vinaigrette, and ½ tbsp olive oil. Salt and pepper to taste before serving. Quinoa is a nutritious grain which contains all essential amino acids with healthy fat and a lower carbohydrate level than rice or wheat. Cook extra quinoa and store in the refrigerator.

Quinoa- Spinach Salad

Quinoa 1 cup and toast in a dry pan until it crackles (approximately 5 minutes), then rinse. Heat 2 tbsp of olive oil and brown 2 tsp minced garlic. Add the Quinoa to the mixture along with 2 cups of water and ½ tsp of salt. Bring to a boil and then decrease the heat and simmer uncovered for 15- 18 minutes (until the water is absorbed). Toss with 1/3 cup of special lemon dressing (see below) and cool for 10 minutes. Add 1 cup halved grape tomatoes and 1 small chopped red onion and toss the mixture. Toss the remaining 1/3 dressing with baby spinach and serve the quinoa mixture over the spinach. Consider topping with toasted almonds or cashews. (Toast in a dry pan).

Special lemon dressing: ¼ cup lemon juice, 2 tbsp non fat plain yogurt, 1 ½ tsp honey, ¼ tsp cumin, ¼ tsp cinnamon, ¼ tsp ginger. Whisk all of the ingredients and then slowly whisk in ¼ cup olive oil. Salt and pepper to taste.

Chopped or Regular Side Salad

Use any combination of Romaine, Boston, Mixed Greens, or Spinach and chop the lettuce or tear the lettuce by hand. Add chopped or sliced cabbage for extra nutrition.

Garnish and toss with any combination of:

- Chopped green onions
- Chopped carrots
- Chopped celery
- Halved grape tomatoes, halved cherry tomatoes, or sliced Roma tomatoes
- Chopped red, yellow, and/or green peppers
- Chopped zucchini
- Chick peas
- Green peas
- Green beans
- Artichoke hearts
- Chopped or whole olives (Green or Kalamata)
- Low fat Feta cheese

Toss with low fat Balsamic vinaigrette dressing or low fat Red Wine vinaigrette dressing. Sprinkle with black pepper.

Side Caesar Salad

Romaine lettuce pieces mixed with halved grape tomatoes. Toss with low fat Caesar dressing and top with low fat Parmesan cheese and sprinkle with black pepper. Add sliced red onion if you wish.

Whole leaf Romaine Side Salad

Use whole leaf romaine lettuce and top with halved grape tomatoes, chopped green onion, and chopped carrots. Drizzle with low fat Balsamic vinaigrette dressing (or low fat Caesar), sprinkle with black pepper, and top with low fat Parmesan cheese.

Sliced Beefsteak Tomato

Slice Beefsteak Tomatoes and drizzle with combination of extra virgin olive oil and balsamic vinegar. Sprinkle with cracked black pepper and a pinch of sea or kosher salt. Add sliced low fat mozzarella cheese if you wish.

Tomato/Onion Side Salad

Combine halved grape tomatoes with sliced red onion and cubed low fat Mozzarella cheese (may cut up the low fat mozzarella snack sticks to save $$). Toss with low fat Balsamic vinaigrette dressing and sprinkle with black pepper and sea or kosher salt. For extra kick toss in seeded chopped Jalapeno peppers.

Applesauce

Use Applesauce cup with no added sugar. Sprinkle with cinnamon for extra flavor. Another quick trick is to add a small amount of low fat maple syrup and sprinkle with cinnamon.

Quick Fruit Salad

Combine ½ oz almonds with diced apples and diced bananas. Mix with 2 tbsp low fat vanilla yogurt. If you wish add diced strawberries and/or halved red grapes.

Broccoli-Red Cabbage Slaw

Combine 12 oz shredded broccoli slaw (or shred fresh broccoli) with 6 oz red cabbage, ½ cup chopped red onion, and 4 slices of cooked center cut bacon or turkey bacon. Toss with the dressing listed below.

Dressing: ¼ cup nonfat plain yogurt, ¼ cup low fat Miracle Whip, 3 tbsp cider vinegar, and 1 tsp sugar (or ½ tsp Splenda sugar product). Whisk ingredients together and salt/pepper to taste.

Quick tip

Fresh vegetables on salads make the nutritional value of the salad superb. Always use low fat vinaigrette based salad dressings. Make your own salad dressing with balsamic or red wine vinegar, olive oil, oregano, basil, parsley, black pepper, garlic, and sea or kosher salt.

Salad dressing options if vinaigrette dressing is not acceptable:

1. Healthy Blue Cheese dressing: ¼ cup crumbled blue cheese, 2 tbsp low fat sour cream, 2 tbsp low fat Miracle Whip, ¼ cup buttermilk, 1 tbsp white wine vinegar, 1 tbsp dried parsley (or fresh chopped), 1 tbsp chopped green onion. Whisk blue cheese, sour cream, and Miracle Whip. Then stir in remaining ingredients. Salt and pepper to taste.
2. Healthy Buttermilk Ranch dressing: ½ cup buttermilk, ¼ cup low fat Miracle Whip, 2 tbsp white wine vinegar, ½ tsp garlic powder, 1/3 cup chopped fresh chives and basil (or 1 tbsp dried basil and 1 tbsp dried chives). Whisk ingredients together. Salt and pepper to taste. Stir in the herbs at the end.

Dinner Recipes

Standard drinks

Water, Caffeine free diet soda, Caffeine free iced tea, Crystal light

---

Grilled or Baked Meat with Herb seasoning

Chicken breast, Turkey breast, Pork loin, or Top Sirloin: 4-8 oz portion (6 oz is an excellent choice) and brush both sides with extra virgin olive oil. Sprinkle with black pepper (or pepper blend), garlic powder (or roasted garlic), onion powder, and sea or kosher salt. Then grill or bake until done. Be sure to fully cook chicken, turkey, and pork to prevent food related infections.

- Option 2: Sprinkle with **garlic powder (or roasted garlic), rosemary, and thyme**
- Option 3: Sprinkle with **crushed red pepper, oregano, sea salt**
- Option 4: **Premade rub** from the grocery store
- Option 5: Top with **Tomato salsa or Mango salsa**
- Option 6: Top with a mixture of 2 tbsp **low sodium soy sauce**, 2 tbsp **low fat maple syrup**, and ¼ tsp of **cracked red pepper**. Wisk ingredients together before using as a topping

Sides: Vegetable of choice and side salad of choice.

Quick tip

When grilling, wipe the grill grate with extra virgin olive oil or spray with a heat resistant vegetable spray. This will prevent sticking and improved the char-grilled lines on the item. For fun with fish, rotate the serving 90 degrees during the grilling process to create crossed grill lines like you see at a restaurant.

Grilled or Baked Fish with Herb seasoning

Salmon, Tilapia, or Orange Roughy. All of these fish are available fresh (actually previously frozen unless you buy it from the fisherman) or frozen. 4-8 oz portion (6 oz is and excellent choice) and brush both sides with extra virgin olive oil. Sprinkle with black pepper or pepper blend, garlic powder, onion powder, and sea salt. Then grill or bake until done.

- Option 2: Sprinkle with **black pepper, sea or kosher salt, rosemary, and thyme**
- Option 3. Sprinkle with **crushed red pepper, oregano, and sea or kosher salt**
- Option 4: Premade rub from the grocery store (**Old Bay Seasoning or Everglades Seasoning) with sea or kosher salt**
- Option 5: Top with **Tomato salsa or Mango salsa**
- Option 6: Top with a mixture of 2 tbsp **low salt soy sauce (Kikoman's)**, 2 tbsp **low fat maple syrup**, and ¼ tsp **cracked red pepper**

Sides: Vegetable of choice with a side salad of choice.

Grilled Shrimp or Sea Scallops with Herb seasoning

Large shrimp or sea scallops and brush with extra virgin olive oil. Sprinkle with black pepper, garlic powder, onion powder, and sea salt. May also sauté in a pan coated with Pam or a small amount of extra virgin olive oil.

- Option 2: Sprinkle with **Old Bay Seasoning**
- Option 3: Sprinkle with **Everglades seasoning**
- Option 4: Sprinkle with **pepper, rosemary, thyme**
- Option 5: Top with **Tomato salsa or Mango salsa**
- Option 6: Top with a mixture of 2 tbsp **low sodium soy sauce**, 2 tbsp **low fat maple syrup**, and ¼ tsp **cracked red pepper**

Sides: Vegetable of choice and side salad of choice.

Quick tip

If using wooden skewers, soak the skewers in water for 30 minutes before using. This will prevent burning of the wood on the grill. When grilling shrimp place the shrimp very close together on the skewer as this will help prevent excessive drying of the shrimp during the grilling time.

Grilled Hamburger/Cheeseburger

Use 92-95% lean beef. Brush with extra virgin olive oil then sprinkle with roasted garlic (or garlic powder), pepper blend (or black pepper), sea salt, and splash with Worcestershire sauce. When grilling, melt low fat American cheese or low fat Jarlsberg cheese on the burger. Top with tomato, lettuce, and pickle if you wish. Add any combination of mustard, catsup, and low fat Miracle Whip. You may also consider topping the burger with salsa. Be sure to use a whole wheat hamburger bun or no bun at all.

- **Healthy option**: Change to a **Turkey burger** or **Vege burger** (Boca burger) and season as above
- **Special burger**: Mix meat with chopped red or sweet onion, chopped fresh spinach, and 2 tbsp oats. Then garnish as above
- **Salmon burger**: Canned salmon flaked with a fork. Add minced garlic, parsley, finely chopped sweet or red onion, pepper, sea salt, and 1 tbsp Worcestershire sauce. Top with low fat Miracle Whip

Sides: Vegetable of choice and banana stuffed with peanut butter, then sliced

---

Shish Kebob

Any combination of cubed Chicken, cubed Top Sirloin, and/or Shrimp. Marinate in fat free or low fat Italian dressing. Place the meat on a skewer with sweet or red onion, red and/or green bell pepper, pineapple, mushrooms, and zucchini. Brush with fat free or low fat Italian dressing and sprinkle with black pepper. Then grill until done. Using precooked chicken or partially cooking the chicken in a microwave after marinating will insure the chicken will be completely done without overcooking the other items on the skewer.

Sides: Applesauce cup with whole wheat roll and low fat butter.

Sea Scallops

Sauté 4 large sea scallops in a pan with extra virgin olive oil. Cook 3 minutes per side on a high heat. Add to the sauté fresh spinach, sliced mushrooms, and chopped green onion. Sprinkle with pepper blend, sea or kosher salt, and garlic powder.

Sides: Tomato/Onion side salad with toasted whole wheat English muffin.

Baked Sea Scallops

Wrap 4 large sea scallops in aluminum foil with thin sliced sweet onion, sliced carrots, and sliced red peppers. Drizzle with extra virgin olive oil and sprinkle with sea or kosher salt and black pepper. Bake at 400 degrees for 12 minutes. Open and add premade Pesto sauce.

Sides: Vegetable of choice and side salad.

Chopped or Regular Dinner Salad with Chicken and/or Shrimp

Use any mixture of chopped or hand torn Romaine lettuce, Boston lettuce, and/or Spinach.

Garnish and toss with any combination of:

- Chopped carrots- very nutritious
- Broccoli florets- small- best of the best in the vegetable nutritious world
- Chopped green onions
- Chopped mushrooms
- Chopped red, yellow, or green peppers- very important
- Chopped celery
- Halved grape tomatoes- very important
- Chopped zucchini- great to create a full feeling along with nutrition
- Artichoke hearts
- Chick peas- very important for protein and fiber
- Green peas- excellent protein
- Green beans- excellent protein
- Chopped or whole green olives or kalamata olives- excellent unsaturated fat addition
- Low fat Feta cheese

- Precooked chicken or shrimp

Toss with low fat Balsamic vinaigrette dressing or Red Wine vinaigrette dressing. Top with black pepper. May add low fat Parmesan cheese if you wish (do not use with Feta cheese).

> Sides: One half whole wheat bagel or whole wheat roll with a smear of low fat butter. Sprinkle with garlic powder and paprika and toast in the oven.

Quick tip

Fresh dressing option: 1 tbsp of Extra Virgin Olive Oil with 3 tbsp of Balsamic or Red wine vinegar (add to your taste). Mix in to taste, garlic powder, oregano, basil, parsley, pepper, and sea or kosher salt. Optimum is to use chopped fresh oregano, basil, and parsley. Use a whisk blending method, stick blender, or salad blender to mix the ingredients. Increase the olive oil amount if the dressing tastes too much like vinegar.

Apple/Lettuce Dinner Salad with Chicken and/or Shrimp

Combine Boston lettuce with Spinach. Hand tear the leaves or coarsely chop with a knife. Add halved grape tomatoes, sliced carrots, and sliced green onions. Toss in low fat Raspberry vinaigrette or low fat Red wine vinaigrette. Sprinkle with black pepper and low fat Parmesan cheese. Add precooked chicken and/or shrimp. Top with sliced apples (Gala or Fuji are excellent choices).

Sides: One half whole wheat bagel or whole wheat roll with a smear of low fat butter. Sprinkle with garlic powder and paprika and toast in the oven.

Flatbread Pizza

Whole wheat crust or flatbread with toppings. Thin crust whole wheat Boboli, whole wheat pita, or whole wheat thin flatbread also are all excellent options. Brush the crust with extra virgin olive oil, sprinkle with sea salt and garlic powder, add low fat mozzarella cheese and toppings, top with oregano, basil, and black pepper. Then bake 6-10 minutes at 375 degrees. For best results preheat a pizza stone and bake the pizza on this. Consider topping the pizza with crushed red pepper for more zip.

- **Marinara sauce, low fat mozzarella cheese, and low fat Parmesan cheese.** Top with any combination of sliced red or sweet onion, sliced mushrooms, portabella mushroom, sliced red or green pepper, chopped broccoli, precooked shrimp, precooked chicken, low fat ham, Canadian bacon, or precooked shrimp. Be creative with healthy choices.
- **White pizza with low fat mozzarella cheese, low fat Parmesan cheese, and sliced Roma tomatoes.** Add any combination of sliced red onions, sliced mushrooms, sliced red pepper, precooked shrimp, precooked chicken, low fat ham, Canadian bacon, or precooked shrimp.
- **BBQ pizza with BBQ sauce and low fat mozzarella cheese.** Top with diced tomatoes, chopped green onions, chopped chili peppers, and chopped cilantro.
- **Marinara sauce, low fat mozzarella cheese, and low fat Parmesan cheese.** Top with fresh sliced Portobello mushroom, sliced red onion, and fresh leaf Spinach.
- **Marinara sauce with low fat mozzarella cheese and low fat Parmesan cheese.** Top with sliced red onion and turkey pepperoni.

Sides: Side salad of choice and cup of applesauce.

Vegetable Soup Dinner

Combine one 12 oz can low sodium chicken broth (Swanson's is the best for the price), one half can petite diced tomatoes, 1 tsp low fat butter, 1 cup frozen mixed vegetables (or frozen vegetable soup mix), one half cup frozen broccoli, sliced mushrooms, chopped green onion, and any left over vegetables (zucchini, asparagus, etc). Season with black pepper, garlic powder, basil, and oregano. Bring to a boil, then reduce heat and simmer for 30 minutes.

> Sides: Side salad of choice and one whole wheat roll dipped in extra virgin olive oil. Sprinkle the olive oil with black pepper and crushed red pepper.

Chicken Soup Dinner

Combine one 12 oz can low sodium chicken broth (Swanson's is the best for the price), one cup frozen mixed vegetables, one cup precooked chicken (chopped), 1 tsp low fat butter, chopped green onions, chopped celery, and one half cup egg noodles or cubed red potatoes (microwave potatoes first). Season with garlic powder, black pepper, oregano, and basil. Bring to a boil then reduce heat and simmer for 30 minutes.

> Sides: Side salad of choice with whole wheat crackers.

Quick tip

Excellent herb mixture for dipping bread: Combine chopped fresh garlic cloves, chopped fresh parsley, chopped fresh oregano, chopped fresh basil, chopped fresh thyme, crushed black peppercorns, cracked red pepper, and sea or kosher salt. Chop well, mix and serve with a small amount of extra virgin olive oil. This may substitute for low fat butter on any bread product.

Spaghetti

Whole wheat pasta (choice of type) cooked in lightly salted water (Remember whole wheat pasta may take slightly longer to cook). Sauté in extra virgin olive oil lean hamburger or crumbled vege/griller "meat", chopped sweet onion, and chopped mushrooms. Then add ½ jar of premade spaghetti sauce (Bertoli is my favorite) and 1 tsp low fat butter. Season with oregano, garlic powder (or minced garlic), and black pepper. Simmer for 30 minutes before topping the pasta.

 Sides: Vegetable of choice topped with low fat butter mixed with garlic and pepper.

Chicken and/or Shrimp Fried Rice Meal

Sauté/stir fry in extra virgin olive oil a combination of sliced carrots, chopped green onions, sliced mushrooms, peas, green beans, and broccoli. Add one half cup of low sodium chicken broth and bring to a boil. Transfer to a holding bowl and scramble one egg. Add back the vegetables and add two cups of cooked brown rice. Season with low sodium Soy sauce (Kikoman's is the best).

 Sides: Egg drop soup. Bring remaining chicken broth to a boil and add one uncooked beaten egg (use a whipping brush), peas, chopped green onion, and ½ tsp corn starch. Season with black pepper, garlic powder, and basil. Simmer for 15 minutes mixing with a whipping brush frequently.

Steak, Chicken, Shrimp, and/or Portobello mushroom Fajitas

Use any combination of steak, chicken, shrimp, and/or Portobello mushroom and marinade in 2 tbsp lime juice, 1 tsp chili powder, and a pinch of crushed red pepper. Shake in a Ziploc bag and drain the residual marinade after 30 minutes. Sauté in extra virgin olive oil sliced red peppers, sliced sweet onions, and the "meat." Wrap in warmed whole wheat tortillas and add salsa (or pico de gallo) and fat free sour cream. May add guacamole and/or chopped lettuce if you wish. For guacamole take one ripe guacamole, half and remove the pit. Then scope out the inside and mash with a fork. Add minced garlic, chopped Roma tomatoes, chopped red onion, chopped jalapeno peppers, and chopped Cilantro. Salt and pepper to taste, mix and serve.

- Option 1: Toss in a premade fajitas marinade.
- Option 2: Special Texas Marinade: combine ½ cup water, ½ cup soy sauce, ½ cup white vinegar, ½ cup olive oil, 1 tbsp minced dry onion, 1 tsp oregano, ¼ tsp black pepper, and ¼ tsp crushed red pepper. Best flavor if marinated overnight but 30 minutes is the short version.

Sides: Corn on the cob and baked tortilla chips with salsa.

Chili

Meat or Meatless: Brown ½ pound of low fat hamburger or an 8-12 oz package of frozen soy protein crumbles. Then combine in a crock pot the meat or soy, one onion finely chopped, ½ green or red bell pepper chopped and seeded, 1 stick celery chopped, 1 carrot finely chopped, 2 tbsp minced garlic, two Jalapeno peppers chopped and seeded, one half cup water, 2 tsp chili powder, 2 tsp oregano, 1 tsp cumin, ¾ tsp sea salt, one 28 oz can crushed tomatoes, and one 15 ½ oz can red kidney beans (rinsed and drained). For extra tomato flavor add one 15 oz can of diced tomatoes. Add chopped zucchini or chopped cilantro if you have extra in the fridge. Simmer for 4 hours in a crock pot or on the stove. If you wish, top with fat free sour cream and/or chopped green onions.

Sides: One whole wheat roll with low fat butter or fresh herb dipping mix. Add a side salad of choice.

Navy Bean Soup with Grilled Cheese Sandwich

Grilled cheese sandwich: Whole wheat bread with low fat butter spread on one side of each slice, add low fat American or low fat Sharp Cheddar cheese, spray a pan with vegetable spray, then grill. Navy bean soup: In a medium saucepan sauté minced garlic in extra virgin olive oil. Add one 15oz can of Navy beans rinsed and drained, one half cup dried parsley, 2 tbsp lemon juice, 4 tsp dried rosemary, ½ tsp ground black pepper, ½ tsp sea or kosher salt, and 2 cups low sodium chicken broth. Bring to a boil and then simmer for 15 minutes.

Sides: Applesauce cup.

Maryland Crab Cakes

One half pound cooked lump crab meat combined with ½ cup whole wheat bread crumbs, 1 chopped green onion or shallot, 1/8 cup skim milk, 1 ½ tbsp Miracle Whip, ½ tsp Old Bay Seasoning, 1/8 tsp white pepper, a pinch of sea or kosher salt, and half an egg, beaten. Mix and form into 4 crab cakes then refrigerate one hour. Remove from refrigerator and cover each side with flour (or even better almond or chick pea flour). Sauté in melted low fat butter on medium high heat, 4-5 minutes on each side. Serve with tarter sauce made with low fat Miracle Whip dressing. (2 tbsp of Miracle Whip, 1 tbsp HFCA free catsup, 1 tsp of relish).

- **Special sauce:** Combine in a bowl ½ cup low fat Miracle Whip, 1 tsp Dijon mustard, 1 tsp minced garlic, 1 ½ tsp sweet pickle relish, 1 tsp lemon juice, 1 tsp minced parsley, salt, and black pepper. Placed the mixture in a food processor and pulse blend for 5 seconds.

Sides: Side salad of choice and cup of applesauce.

Snow Crab Legs

Steam for 8 minutes and serve with melted low fat butter. May substitute King crab legs or when available Stone crab claws.

Sides: Broccoli and Corn on the cob. One whole wheat roll with low fat butter (or fresh herb dipping mix).

Sautéed Shrimp with Broccoli and Peas

Shrimp, Broccoli, Peas, Lemon, and Green Onions. Melt 2 tbsp of low fat butter in a large skillet. Sauté broccoli, white part of chopped green onions, lemon zest, and small amount of water. Season with salt and pepper. Cover and cook 3-4 minutes until broccoli is done. Add shrimp and peas and cook until peas are tender and shrimp is done. Add 2 tbsp of lemon juice, the green part of the green onions, 1 tbsp of low fat butter, additional salt and pepper. Toss gently then serve.

Sides: Side chopped salad.

Shrimp Salad stuffed Tomato

Combine ½ lb chopped cooked shrimp with ½ stalk chopped celery, 5 chopped Kalamata or Green olives, 1 small chopped shallot, 1 tbsp low fat Miracle Whip, and ½ tsp white wine vinegar. Season to taste with black pepper. Core out 2 large tomatoes and stuff with the shrimp salad. This is a great dinner when tomatoes are in season.

Side: Steamed asparagus or steamed broccoli.

Whole wheat Penne with Grape Tomatoes, Chick peas, and Mozzarella cubes

Boil whole wheat penne in water salted with sea salt. Reserve a small amount of the water in a cup. Add chick peas (8-15 oz depending on amount of pasta) and drain pasta/chick pea mixture. Return the mixture to the pot and add halved grape tomatoes, low fat mozzarella cheese cubed, 2 tbsp of thyme, 1 tbsp of white wine vinegar, and 2 tbsp of olive oil. Toss together using the reserve pasta water in small amounts to create a sauce and coat the penne. Season with sea salt and pepper, toss again, top with parsley, and serve.

Sides: Broccoli and whole wheat roll with low fat butter.

Quick Dinners

Frozen Healthy Choice or Lean Cuisine dinners both have many excellent choices with constant new ideas. Reference the frozen food recommendations in this book.

Sides: Side salad of choice.

Quick tip

Remember to emphasize vegetables as your carbohydrate in the evening with fruit carbs earlier in the day. A small amount of whole wheat carbs in the evening is acceptable as this will decrease your cravings.

Part IV

Specific Nutritional Considerations

Fast Foods: Acceptable Options

Fast foods are never the first choice for a healthy diet, but are a fact of life. Many times we need to eat quickly and do not have time to make a nutritious meal at home or sit down to a reasonably nutritious meal at a restaurant. Subway has clearly worked hard to offer an acceptably healthy fast food meal. Other options are much worse but if you are careful and watch the portions fast foods can be an acceptable occasional option. The following presents the best choices from representative fast foods.

Quick tip

Remember to always eat the appropriate foods over the course of the day.

Do not obsess about calories but in this review the nutritional value is provided for these fast foods for comparison information.

❖ Indicates the best choices

Arbys

❖ **Hot Ham and Swiss Melt**

270Kcal/ 18grams protein/ 35grams carbs/ 8grams fat/ 3.5grams saturated fat/ 35mg cholesterol/ 1gram fiber/ 1140mg sodium

▪ **Jr. Roast Beef**

270Kcal/ 16grams protein/ 34grams carbs/ 9grams fat/ 4grams saturated fat/ 30mg cholesterol/ 2grams fiber/ 740mg sodium

- **Martha's Vineyard Market Fresh Salad- no dressing**

  250Kcal/ 26grams protein/ 23grams carbs/ 8grams fat/ 4.5grams saturated fats/ 60mg cholesterol/ 4grams fiber/ 490mg sodium—will need to add salad dressing and adjust figures based on the dressing

Quick tip

Sodium (salt) content is high in essentially all fast foods.

Burger King

- **Tendergrill Chicken Sandwich**

  450Kcal/ 37grams protein/ 10grams fat/ 2grams saturated fat/ 75mg cholesterol/ 4grams fiber/ 1210mg sodium

- **Tendergrill Chicken Filet Salad**

  420Kcal/ 35grams protein/ 23grams carbs/ 22grams fat/ 6grams saturated fat/ 80mg cholesterol/ 5grams fiber/ 1280mg sodium (11grams of fat in the dressing despite light Italian)

Quick tip

Choices overall quite poor at Burger King so be careful.

Domino's

❖ **Classic Hand Tossed Pepperoni- one slice**

200Kcal/ 8grams protein/ 28grams carbs/ 6.5grams fat/ 2grams saturated fat/ 5mg cholesterol/ 1gram fiber/ 250mg sodium—add vegetables without any significant additional calories

Cheese slice with very similar nutritional figures

▪ **Vegi Feast Crunch Thin Crust**

231Kcal/ 10grams protein/ 21grams carbs/ 13.5grams fat/ 5gram saturated fat/ 19mg cholesterol/ 2grams fiber/ 551mg sodium

Hardees

❖ **Slammer**

240Kcal/ 13grams protein/ 19grams carbs/ 12grams fat/ 5gram saturated fats/ 35mg cholesterol/ 0grams fiber/ 300mg sodium

▪ **Regular Roast Beef Sandwich**

330Kcal/ 19grams protein/ 29grams carbs/ 16grams fat/ 7grams saturated fat/ 40mg cholesterol/ 2grams fiber/ 860mg sodium

Little Caesars

❖ **Thin Crust Pepperoni or Cheese Pizza- one slice**

210Kcal/ 11grams protein/ 23grams carbs/ 7.6grams fat/ 4grams saturated fat/ 20mg cholesterol/ 400mg sodium—add vegetables without much increase in calories

- **Deep Dish Cheese Pizza- one slice**

  230Kcal/ 11grams protein/ 27grams carbs/ 9.2grams fat/ 4grams saturated fat/ 15mg cholesterol/ 1gram fiber/ 340mg sodium

Quick tip

One slice of pizza is an acceptable fast food. Try to load up on the vegetables to supply a filling and satisfying meal.

McDonalds

- ❖ **Grilled Chicken Caesar Salad with low fat Balsamic Vinaigrette Dressing**

  240Kcal/ 29grams protein/ 13grams carbs/ 9grams fat/ 3grams saturated fat/ 70mg cholesterol/ 3grams fiber/ 1550mg sodium

- **Chicken McGrill- no mayo- add mustard for flavor**

  300Kcal/ 27grams protein/ 37grams carbs/ 4.5grams fat/ 1gram saturated fat/ 60mg cholesterol/ 3gram fiber/ 940mg sodium

- **Hamburger**

  280Kcal/ 12grams protein/ 36grams carbs/ 10grams fat/ 4grams saturated fats/ 30mg cholesterol/ 2grams fiber/ 550mg sodium

Papa Johns

❖ **Garden Fresh Original Crust Pizza- one slice**

270Kcal/ 40grams carbs/ 9grams fat/ 2.5grams saturated fat/ 10mg cholesterol/ 2grams fiber/ 680mg sodium

▪ **Cheese Original Crust Pizza- one slice**

300Kcal/ 13grams protein/ 39grams carbs/ 11grams fat/ 3.5grams saturated fat/ 20mg cholesterol/ 2grams fiber/ 770mg sodium—add vegetables!!

▪ **Pepperoni Original Crust Pizza- one slice**

330Kcal/ 14grams protein/ 39grams carbs/ 14grams fat/ 4.5grams saturated fat/ 25mg cholesterol/ 2grams fiber/ 860mg sodium—add vegetables!!

Pizza Hut

❖ **Fit'n Delicious Pizza- with Green Pepper, Red Onion, and Tomatoes- one slice**

140Kcal/ 6grams protein/ 22grams carbs/ 4grams fat/ 1.5grams saturated fat/ 10mg cholesterol/ 2grams fiber/ 330mg sodium

❖ **Fit'n Delicious Pizza- with Ham, Red Onion, and Mushroom- one slice**

150Kcal/ 8grams protein/ 21grams carbs/ 4grams fat/ 2grams saturated fat/ 15mg cholesterol/ 2grams fiber/ 440mg sodium

▪ **Pepperoni Hand Tossed Pizza- one slice**

240Kcal/ 12grams protein/ 27grams carbs/ 11grams fat/ 4.5grams saturated fat/ 1gram trans fat/ 25mg cholesterol/ 1gram fiber/ 640mg sodium

Quick tip

Watch for trans fat in fast foods and they are worse than saturated fat. The "new" trans fat is esterified fats so watch carefully for these. Avoid all trans and esterified fats.

Subway- clearly the best!!!

❖ **Turkey Breast Sub- 6 inches**

210Kcal/ 13grams protein/ 36grams carbs/ 3.5grams fat/ 1.5grams saturated fat/ 15mg cholesterol/ 3grams fiber/ 730mg sodium

❖ **Ham Deli Sub- 6 inches**

210Kcal/ 11grams protein/ 35grams carbs/ 4grams fat/ 1.5grams saturated fat/ 10mg cholesterol/ 3grams fiber/ 770mg sodium

❖ **Vege Delite Sub- 6 inches**

230Kcal/ 9grams protein/ 44grams carbs/ 3grams fat/ 1gram saturated fat/ 0mg cholesterol/ 4grams fiber/ 510mg sodium

Quick tip

Overall there are excellent choices at Subway. Be sure to change whole wheat sub roll or wrap to maximize the good carbs. The subs are still moderately high in sodium so do not add extra salt.

Taco Bell

❖ **Taco Supreme- Fresco Style**

150Kcal/ 7grams protein/ 15grams carbs/ 7grams fat/ 2.5grams saturated fat/ 20mg cholesterol/ 2grams fiber/ 360mg sodium

❖ **Tostada- Fresco Style**

200Kcal/ 8grams protein/ 30grams carbs/ 6grams fat/ 1gram saturated fat/ 0mg cholesterol/ 8grams fiber/ 670mg sodium

▪ **Chicken Gordita Supreme - Fresco Style**

230Kcal/ 15grams protein/ 28grams carbs/ 6grams fat/ 1gram saturated fat/ 25mg cholesterol/ 2grams fiber/ 1040mg sodium

▪ **Chicken Burrito Supreme- Fresco Style**

350Kcal/ 19grams protein/ 50grams carbs/ 8grams fat/ 2grams saturated fat/ 1.5grams transfat/ 25mg cholesterol/ 6grams fiber/ 1270mg sodium

Quick tip

Fresco style is a Fiesta Salsa substituted for the cheese and/or sauce.

Wendy's

- **Jr. Hamburger**

  270Kcal/ 15grams protein/ 34grams carbs/ 9grams fat/ 3.5grams saturated fat/ 30mg cholesterol/ 2grams fiber/ 610mg sodium

- **Ultimate Chicken Grill**

  360Kcal/ 31grams protein/ 44grams carbs/ 8grams fat/ 1.5grams saturated fat/ 75mg cholesterol/ 2grams fiber/ 1100mg sodium

- **Cranberry Peca Chicken Salad with Berry Balsamic Vinaigrette**

  350Kcal/ 23grams protein/ 42grams carbs/ 10grams fat/ 1.5grams saturated fat/ 60mg cholesterol/ 5grams fiber

- **Frescata Turkey and Basil Pesto**

  420Kcal/ 23grams protein/ 50grams carbs/ 15grams fat/ 3grams saturated fat/ 40mg cholesterol/ 4grams fiber

Moes

- ❖ **The Full Monty Chicken Soft Taco**

  210Kcal/ 14grams protein/ 19grams carbs/ 8grams fat/ 4grams saturated fat/ 34mg cholesterol/ 5grams fiber/ 525mg sodium

- **The Other Lewinsky Soft Taco- (with sour cream and guacamole)**

282Kcal/ 14grams protein/ 21grams carbs/ 15grams fat/ 8grams saturated fat/ 54mg cholesterol/ 5grams fiber/ 717mg sodium

- **Joey Bag of Donuts- streaker (without tortilla)**

  463 Kcal/ 48grams carbs/17grams fat/ 8grams saturated fat/ 67mg cholesterol/ 7grams fiber/ 1327mg sodium

Quick tip

Fast foods are generally a poor choice but are commonly a necessity in our busy lifestyle. Minimize their intake for a healthy lifestyle. Subway is the overall fast food winner for the best nutritional value. Watch the fast food menu's as they are constantly changing with an increased attention to healthier options.

Restaurant Dining

Many restaurants have realized their patrons are starting to understand that nutrition is one of the keys to healthy living. There are now many restaurants that include menu sections which contain foods choices for a healthy meal. Even without these sections there are methods which improve the nutritional value of the meal when ordering off the regular menu. When eating out the one problem which is the hardest to overcome is the amount of salt added to restaurant food. Usually it is excessive and difficult to minimize. High fat meals can quickly be improved by changing the side item to a steamed vegetable.

Quick restaurant rules:

- Best entrees are grilled, baked, broiled, or steamed. Avoid breaded, fried, and deep fried foods.
- Eat small portions- set a portion off to the side before you start eating and take the left over's home for lunch or a snack.
- Consider ordering from the appetizer menu for your main dish. Smaller portions and still excellent taste.
- Change potatoes/French fries or rice to a side of steamed vegetables.
- If ordering rice change to brown rice.
- If ordering bread change to whole wheat, sourdough, pumpernickel, or rye.
- Order salad dressings on the side and change to a vinaigrette type dressing. Even better, take a small container of low fat oil based dressing with you.
- Cut off excess fat from meat and remove the skin from the chicken.
- Choose red or marinara sauce over the cream based white or fettuccini sauce.
- Eat slowly as this will allow your brain to inform your body that you are full.
- Avoid regular soda as this is pure empty calories. If in doubt drink water.
- Avoid foods labeled with au gratin, au lait, creamed, and a la mode due to the high calorie cream base.
- Do not miss scheduled snacks. Without the snacks you will be excessively hungry at meal time and will overeat.
- Ask the restaurant for special requests if you do not see a healthy choice.
- Use low fat or skim milk for your coffee.

- Avoid dessert.

Best Breakfast options:

- **Eat at home: Start the day nutritionally correct!!!**
- **On the go breakfast:** Reasonable second choice.
    - ✓ ½ whole wheat English muffin with peanut butter and topped with sliced apple.
    - ✓ Light and Fit French Vanilla Yogurt (flavored or add sliced/chopped fresh fruit or blend with frozen mixed fruit). For extra crunch top with low fat granola.
    - ✓ Light and Fit Strawberry Banana Smoothie.
    - ✓ Low fat cottage cheese topped with sliced or chopped fresh fruit.
    - ✓ Breakfast bars: Special K, Fiber One (Oats and Chocolate), Cascadian farm organic, or Kashi TLC.
- **Breakfast restaurant:**
    - ✓ Cereal (Cheerios, Special K, Shredded Wheat) with skim milk and topped with sliced fruit or a side of fresh fruit.
    - ✓ Oatmeal (careful with the brown sugar topping).
    - ✓ Eggs (or substitute egg beater) with Canadian bacon and whole wheat toast or whole wheat English muffin.
    - ✓ Eggs (or substitute egg beater) with fresh fruit side.
    - ✓ Spinach and feta cheese omelet is generally a good choice.
    - ✓ Always order whole wheat toast or whole wheat English muffin.
    - ✓ Unhealthy choices include pancakes, sausage, home fries, muffins, and sticky buns.
- **Fast food:** Mediocre choices overall.
    - ✓ Egg McMuffin (with or without Canadian bacon). **Best quick choice.** If available whole wheat English muffin. Add a slice of tomato for extra nutrition.
    - ✓ Chicken biscuit but try to exchange the biscuit for an English muffin (whole wheat if available). Add a slice of tomato for extra nutrition.

Best Lunch options:

- **Subway, Blimpies, or Quizno's subs or wraps**: Ask for whole wheat bread or whole wheat wrap. Avoid adding high calorie mayo or special sauces. Stick to mustard, low fat mayo, and olive oil/vinegar as dressings. Add multiple vegetables and keep the cheese to a minimum. Side dishes with baked chips, low fat yogurt, or fruit.
- **Fast food**: See outlined options in the fast food section.
- **Boston Market**: Chicken or Turkey (skinless and white meat) with sides of steamed vegetables. Avoid the pasta sides and careful with the corn bread.
- **Chili's/Applebee's/TGI Friday's/etc**: As outlined in the dinner section.
- **Atlanta Bread Company**:
  - ✓ Roasted Turkey Breast on Nine Grain bread. Dress with mustard.
- **Panera**:
  - ✓ BBQ Chicken Crispani.
  - ✓ Low fat Vegetarian Garden Vegetable Soup with whole grain bread.
- **Chipotle**:
  - ✓ Chicken Burrito Bowl with lettuce, black beans, green tomatilio salsa, and sour cream.
  - ✓ Crispy Steak Tacos with corn salsa, red tomatilio salsa, and romaine lettuce.
- **Fazoli's**:
  - ✓ Chicken and Fruit Salad with fat free honey mustard dressing.
  - ✓ Small Penne with Marinara and topped with grilled chicken or shrimp, and broccoli. Side salad with fat free Italian dressing.
- **On the Border**:
  - ✓ Chicken Salsa Fresca with grilled vegetables and black bean and corn relish.
- **Panda Express**:
  - ✓ Broccoli beef with mixed vegetables.
  - ✓ String Bean Chicken Breast with mixed vegetables.
  - ✓ Mushroom Chicken with mixed vegetables.
  - ✓ Avoid the rice and noodles.
- **Schlotzsky's**:
  - ✓ Small Smoked Turkey Breast Sandwich.
  - ✓ Fresh Tomato and Pesto Pizza.
  - ✓ Mediterranean Tuna Wrap.

- ✓ Hearty Vegetable Beef Soup and Side Salad with vinaigrette dressing.
- **Uno Chicago Grill:**
  - ✓ Cheese and Tomato Flatbread Pizza. Add fresh vegetables for extra flavor.
  - ✓ BBQ Grilled Shrimp.
  - ✓ Always order the flatbread pizza and avoid the deep dish pizza.
- **Sandwich shop**: Avoid special sauces on the sandwiches. Stick to low fat lunch meats, careful with the cheese, load up on vegetables, and use mustard or low fat mayo or olive oil/vinegar. Choose the baked chip products or fruit as a side.

Quick tip

Appropriate drinks with lunch or dinner include water, iced tea (preferably caffeine free), diet soda (again caffeine free). It is imperative to avoid regular soda as this is pure empty calories.

Dinner options:

- **Chili's:**
  - ✓ Guiltless menu is the first choice.
  - ✓ Chicken fajita pita.
  - ✓ Sizzle and Spice Firecracker Tilapia.
- **Applebee's:**
  - ✓ Weight watcher menu is the first choice.
  - ✓ Teriyaki Steak and Shrimp Skewers.
  - ✓ Grilled Cajun Lime Tilapia.
- **TGI Fridays:**
  - ✓ Healthy section is the first choice.
  - ✓ Sizzling Chicken with Broccoli side.
- **Ruby Tuesday's:**
  - ✓ Salad bar with vinaigrette dressing.

- ✓ Top sirloin with baby green beans.
- ✓ Grilled chicken with baby green beans.
- ✓ White Bean Chicken Chili.

- **Outback/Longhorn's/ and other Steak houses**:
  - ✓ Top sirloin or Filet with vegetable side.
  - ✓ Grilled chicken with vegetable side.
  - ✓ Grilled fish- salmon or tilapia with vegetable side.
  - ✓ Grilled shrimp with vegetable side.
  - ✓ Change the potato/pasta to an additional steamed vegetable.
  - ✓ Use vinaigrette dressings on the salad (or bring from home a small cup of your favorite healthy dressing).
  - ✓ Bread preferences are whole wheat, sourdough, or pumpernickel.

- **Carrabba's Italian**:
  - ✓ Top sirloin grilled with vegetable side.
  - ✓ Grilled chicken with vegetable side.
  - ✓ Grilled fish or shrimp with vegetable side.
  - ✓ Half order of Chicken parmesan with vegetable side.
  - ✓ Pasta entrée use the marinara sauce and not a cream based sauce.
  - ✓ Vinaigrette dressing on the salad.
  - ✓ Minimize the bread intake although the olive oil/herb dipping sauce is excellent.

- **Italian restaurants**:
  - ✓ Pasta entrée's with marinara sauce and a side of steamed vegetables. Avoid the cream based sauces.
  - ✓ Grilled top sirloin, chicken, fish, shrimp with vegetable side.
  - ✓ Chicken parmesan with vegetable side. (Cut in half and take home the extra).
  - ✓ Vinaigrette dressing on the salad.
  - ✓ Careful with the garlic bread intake.

- **Crispers/Sweet Tomato/salad based restaurant**:
  - ✓ Darker green lettuce, spinach, and load up on the vegetables. Use a vinaigrette based dressing.
  - ✓ Avoid the cream based soups.
  - ✓ Fresh fruit.
  - ✓ Sandwiches use whole wheat or sourdough bread/wrap with low fat meat, add vegetables, and dress with mustard or olive oil/vinegar.

- **P.F. Chang's:**
  - ✓ Ginger Chicken and Broccoli.
  - ✓ Seared Ahi Tuna.
  - ✓ Wild Alaskan Sockeye.
  - ✓ Order brown rice or skip the rice.
- **Red Lobster:**
  - ✓ Live Maine Lobster with broccoli. Careful with the dipping butter as this will quickly add calories.
  - ✓ Broiled Flounder with broccoli.
  - ✓ Garlic Grilled Jumbo Shrimp with broccoli.
- **High end restaurants: Enjoy your dinner and eat nutritious tomorrow!!!**
- **Creekside Eatery at the Crooked Creek Saloon:** Quick plug for a great restaurant in Fraser, Colorado near the Winter Park Ski Resort. Great food with a healthy menu designed for people on vacation trying to watch their caloric intake.

Quick tip

Don't forget your snacks earlier in the day so you do not over eat when you are out for dinner. Take home part of your meal for another snack or meal later.

Performance and Competitive Sports Nutrition

Performance and Competitive sports include multiple levels of activity and competition. From the children's sports programs to adult level competition to college sports all the way to the professional level, nutrition and hydration are crucial to optimal performance. Endurance athletic events are particularly prone to nutritional related problems. **"Hitting the wall"** is a very real phenomenon and occurs when muscles become depleted in glycogen. The result is a complete loss of energy for muscle contraction and the participant is unable to run or move appropriately. Heat exhaustion, and worse yet Heat Stroke, are potential problems related to hydration. In **Heat Exhaustion** the athlete becomes severely dehydrated (volume depleted) and the skin will be cold and clammy with profuse sweating. Immediate treatment involves placing the person in a shaded area and pushing oral fluids or if available IV fluids. **Heat Stroke** is quite different and results in a dry, hot skin without any significant sweating. This is a **medical emergency** as the core body temperature may go above 108 degrees Fahrenheit. Once the event occurs, push oral or IV fluids, place the patient in a shady location, and transport urgently to a medical facility. The optimal method for treating these problems is preventative care with correct nutrition and hydration pre/during/post competition.

Quick tip

Warning: If you are thirsty you are already dehydrated. Drink fluids early and frequently.

Your performance is impaired when you are dehydrated.

The hotter the day and the longer the competition, the more you need to hydrate before, during, and after the competition.

Hydration Guidelines

- ❖ Cold fluids are the best: Refrigerator temperature.
- ❖ When in doubt: Hydrate.
- ▪ Hydrate well the entire day before the event.
- ▪ Drink 24-32 ounces of fluid the night before.
- ▪ Drink 12-16 ounces of fluid early on game day.
- ▪ Drink 8-12 ounces 15 to 30 minutes before the game.
- ▪ During the game drink 4-8 ounces every 20 minutes.
- ▪ Water or Sports drink are equally acceptable. You may consider diluting a sports drink 50:50 with water. My personal preference is Gatorade.
- ▪ **Avoid carbonated beverages**: You will drink less and feel full.
- ▪ **Avoid caffeine**: It is a diuretic and causes fluid loss by increasing urination.
- ▪ Try new beverages in practice first. Do not experiment with new drinks during a game.

Nutritional Recommendations

Quick tip

It is crucial to have appropriate carbohydrate loading before competitive sporting events and even on a constant basis during pre-season training and the regular season. Carbs include pasta, bread, fruits, and vegetables.

Night before the game

Every athlete requires carbohydrate loading the evening before the game. This will help maximize your muscle glycogen stores and improve performance.

Avoiding excess fat at this time is important as fat slows down intestinal contractions. This will decrease performance at game time as there will be extra fluids/food in the intestines due to the slower motility. Carbohydrate loading recommendations include:

- **Spaghetti with marinara sauce**: One meatball or a small amount of low fat hamburger in the sauce is acceptable but be careful. Marinara or tomato sauce is the optimum choice. Other pasta noodles such as ziti, linguine, macaroni, etc are all equally acceptable.
- **Whole wheat pasta**: This is also an excellent choice topped with marinara or tomato sauce, vegetables, and chicken.
- **Pizza**: For the extra carbohydrates, the best choice is deep dish topped with cheese (optimum is low fat cheese) and vegetable toppings. Avoid excess fatty meat toppings and excess cheese. Add chicken or low fat ham for extra protein but a lower fat content. Thin crust is also acceptable, but does not provide the same amount of carbs.
- **Lasagna**: Once again be careful with the amount of cheese and meat. Add vegetables and chicken for great taste and excellent carbs/ protein without excessive fat. Always try to fix the lasagna with low fat cheese.
- **Calzone/Stromboli**: This has an excellent carbohydrate content and for extra nutrition load up the dish with chicken and vegetables. A marinara or tomato sauce continues to be the best choice. White, creamed based sauces are too high in fat.
- **Rice dishes**: Very beneficial, particularly with vegetables added for carbs and flavor. The best choice is brown rice and wild rice.
- **Breads and noodles**: Use a low fat butter or dip in a small amount of olive oil with cracked black pepper.
- **Vegetables and Legumes**: Overall a fantastic source of healthy carbs. Broccoli, green beans, asparagus, and tomato can be added to any dish or used as a side dish.
- **Fruits**: These are also a superb source of carbs and can be a rapid source of carbohydrates, particularly during breaks in the game. Citrus (oranges), grapes, cantaloupe, bananas, honey dew, apples, pineapple, strawberries. blueberries, and raspberries are all great choices.
- **Pancakes**: Certainly high in carbs, but be cautious with the syrup due to the high fat content. Top the pancakes with fresh fruit instead.
- **Carbohydrate rich desserts**: Low fat frozen yogurt, Fig Newton's, Animal crackers, Juice Pops can all be rapid sources of carbohydrates.

- **Proteins**: Use low fat protein sources such as chicken, turkey, lean beef (92-95% fat free hamburger or top sirloin), pork loin, fish, scallops, and shrimp.

Quick tip

Don't forget to hydrate!!! Drink water and sports drinks!!! When in doubt, hydrate.

It takes 45-90 minutes to process fluids so start early.

Pre Game Meal

This is the final chance to maximize muscle glycogen content with carbohydrate intake. Be extremely careful with fats at this time as fat will **SLOW YOU DOWN** and impair performance. It is best to eat a light meal 2-3 hours before game time, but with careful food intake you can eat even up to 1 hour before. The closer to the competition the meal is ingested the less you should eat. Breakfast recommendations include:

- **Cereal with low fat milk and fruit** (bananas, blueberries, raspberries, etc): Good cereal choices include Cheerios, Total, Special K, Raisin Bran, Wheaties, Rice Krispies, and Kix.
- **Bagel with low fat cream cheese with a side of yogurt.**
- **Pancakes or waffles with fresh fruit topping**: Be very careful with syrup at this time due to the high fat content.
- **Oatmeal with raisins or berries (blueberries, raspberries, or strawberries) and low fat milk.**

- **Center cut Bacon, Turkey bacon and Canadian bacon:** Small amounts may be used to spice up the flavor and add protein. Canadian bacon has the lowest fat content.
- **Turkey or Low Fat Ham Sub or Wrap:** Add vegetables for extra flavor.
- **Scramble wrap:** Scrambled eggs with salsa and low fat shredded cheese in a wrap. Add chopped Cilantro and chopped green onions for extra taste.
- **Fresh Fruit:** Citrus (oranges), grapes, bananas, cantaloupe, honey dew, apples, pineapple, and strawberries. Always a great source of carbohydrates.
- **Nutrition bar:** Be careful with the fat content as many "breakfast bars" contain a significant fat. Pick one with a maximum fat content of 5 grams. Special K Bars do not have any HFCS (high fructose corn syrup) which is fantastic.
- **Running late??** Liquid nutrition is the optimum choice with Carnation Instant Breakfast, orange juice with one glass of low fat milk, or a smoothie made with fresh or frozen fruit.
- **Fast food choice:** An Egg McMuffin or Chicken biscuit without cheese is acceptable. Add a cup of orange juice and fresh fruit bowl.

Quick tip

Avoid High Fructose Corn Syrup as this will causes a rapid insulin release and lowers your blood glucose level rapidly. The sugar in the cells will not have time to be converted to glycogen and more likely will be converted to fat. HFCS does not supply extra energy for competitive sports.

During the game

- ❖ Preventing dehydration is critical!!
- ▪ Fluid requirements are 4-8 ounces of cold fluid (water or sports drink) every 15-20 minutes. The individual athlete needs to determine if water or a sports drink works best for them. A combination may be the answer, particularly at halftime. During the flow of play water is the best option.
- ▪ **Salt tablets may be harmful!!!** Without appropriate water intake simultaneously salt tablets can drive the serum sodium to dangerously high levels. They should be avoided unless prescribed by a physician.
- ▪ Half time carbohydrates can be very beneficial. Excellent choices include citrus (oranges), grapes, and to a smaller degree bananas.
- ▪ Chronic cramps during the games?? You need to be evaluated for potassium and magnesium deficiencies. Consider a banana (or another potassium supplement) and magnesium supplementation (Mag oxide 2 tablets) 2 hours before the game. Pickle juice occasionally works even when the cramps have set in.

Quick tip

Hydrate with water during the game. Sports drinks without carbonation are important before, after, and at potentially at halftime.

After the game

- ❖ Need to replace the carbohydrates lost during the competition.

- Muscles are most receptive to carb refueling during the first two hours after the competition.
- Carbohydrate choices are the same as for carb loading the evening before.

Weekend or Extended Training Rules

- Carbohydrate intake is important on a consistent basis.
- Avoid excess fats and when eating fats unsaturated fats are the best. Minimize saturated fat intake and eliminate trans fat.
- Esterified fats are a new form of trans fat and should be avoided.
- Each night requires carb loading.
- Same pre game suggestions.
- If multiple games are played on the same day, between games is crucial. Light carbohydrate intake with minimal fat. Excellent choices include:
    1. **Turkey or Ham subs with low fat mayo.** Load up on the veges but avoid cheese
    2. **Turkey or Ham wrap** with veges
    3. **Fruit**- oranges/citrus, grapes, bananas, cantaloupe, apples, pineapple, honeydew, strawberries, etc
    4. **Smoothies** are an excellent choice- concentrate on fresh or frozen fruit
    5. **Vegetables-** broccoli, green beans, peppers, onions, mushrooms, cabbage, green lettuce, carrots, etc
    6. **Sports nutrition bars**- make sure you do not choose a high fat bar. Five grams of fat per bar or less
    7. **Cereal or Oatmeal**
- ❖ **NO FAST FOODS**: They are loaded in fat. Subway is an exception.
- After the games refuel with carbs.
- Continue hydration between games: **VERY IMPORTANT!!!**

Quick tip

My favorite smoothie: 1 cup fresh or frozen berries, 1 banana, 2 cups orange juice, 1 tbsp low fat vanilla yogurt. Add ice if you wish to make it slushy. Add whey and casein protein for muscle repair if you wish. Blend thoroughly and enjoy!!

Weight loss

Multiple weight loss plans are available for a person to choose from. Many of these plans work very well initially but the person will commonly gain weight when the diet is completed. The key in maintaining weight loss is to change your eating habits, eat healthy, exercise regularly, and stick to the regiment. This is a lifestyle change and it can be extremely beneficial to your overall health and wellness as weight loss can improve and potentially reverse a multitude of medical problems.

Quick Weight Loss Review: Important details are outlined in this chapter and extensively reviewed in other portions of the book, but for the quick look read the following:

> - **Change your lifestyle and set reasonable goals.**
> - **Forget "Fad diets."** The weight loss is unlikely to last.
> - **Nutrition** is the backbone of weight loss. Correct eating habits and controlling food portions is very important.
> - **Exercise** is the second building block. A regular regimen with aerobic and anaerobic exercise is crucial.
> - Medical evaluation should be done before any exercise program.
> - **Over the Counter supplements** that are my personal favorites include Chromium picolinate, Green tea, Conjugated Linoleic acid (CLA), and Alli. It is very reasonable to supplement your exercise and nutrition regiment with Green tea daily and Chromium picolinate daily. The stacking regimen listed below is also effective.
> - **Physician monitored Pharmaceutical weight loss medications** are acceptable for a short time to get the weight loss started but are not a long term answer.

Basic rules of weight loss

- Long term sustained weight loss is based on changing lifestyle habits.
- Lifestyle changes center around nutrition, correct eating habits, and regular exercise.

- Careful calorie counting is not necessary. Instead focus on eating several times a day in small controlled portions. Consider a **food diary** to track what you are eating each day as this will help you realize when you are overeating. This is a small book where you write down everything that you eat and then you can estimate the number of total calories as many people will be very surprised with how much they eat. In general we underestimate how much we are eating and any calorie estimates should be increased by 25% to obtain a more accurate count.
- Weight loss should be 1-2 lbs per week over an extended time.
- Fad diets without lifestyle change generally result in short term results without long term sustained weight loss.
- Medical evaluation prior to a weight loss program is mandatory. You need to insure there are not any metabolic problems which would be contributing to your weight problem and to obtain medical clearance (particularly heart and lung) for the program.
- Exercise aerobically frequently. This is a major key and for maximum weight loss as you need 6 aerobic sessions per week with a minimum of 30 minutes per day. If you have a sedentary job, consider brief "exercise" periods during the day. This may simply consist of walking to the copy machine, etc. Walk up and down stairs rather than taking the elevator. Studies suggest that fat burning enzymes shut down quickly when you are sitting at a desk.
- Every person will have times during the program when your progress plateau's for 1-2 week periods and there is no significant weight loss. It is crucial to continue the program as the weight loss will return. Consider altering your diet and exercise program for a brief time to stimulate weight loss, and then return to your original plans. Also pay particular attention to your caloric intake during this time as it is easy to slip back into "bad" eating habits.
- Set a reasonable goal that can be attained or you will become frustrated. You can always adjust/improve your goals later.
- Medical/Pharmaceutical treatment for weight loss is only a short term adjunctive therapy and does not substitute for lifestyle changes. It should never be the main line long term treatment.
- Bariatric surgery may be an option for morbid obesity, but once again lifestyle changes must be instituted initially.
- Wellness and overall health is strongly tied to appropriate weight, nutrition, and exercise.

Quick tip

Sustained weight loss centers on lifestyle changes. Set a reasonable, attainable goal. You will ultimately be very happy with the long term results and your health will benefit over the years.

Nutrition keys

- **Eating habits:** Clearly this is the most important key. All meals and snacks should be small portions and the caloric intake is spread out over the course of the day. This will prevent a rapid increase in insulin levels which can push sugar into cells where it is converted to fat. It is very important to have 4-6 small portions daily with breakfast, mid morning snack, lunch, mid afternoon snack, dinner, and potentially a 9PM snack. Avoid overeating at any one setting and control the total calories over the course of the day!! Start healthy with breakfast as this will stimulate your metabolism.

- **Carbohydrates:** Healthy carbs include whole wheat products, fruits, and vegetables. Try to avoid the refined carbohydrates such as sugar, white bread, and white pasta. Concentrate the fruit intake earlier in the day with vegetable intake at any time but particularly in the second half of the day. Think correct carbs rather than low carbs.

- **Protein:** Lean protein is the key. Chicken or turkey (particularly white meat without the skin), fish, top sirloin, low fat hamburger (93% lean or better), scallops, shrimp (slightly higher in cholesterol), pork loin, turkey bacon, legumes (beans, peas, etc), dairy products, and eggs are all excellent choices. Other sources include nuts and soybean which are very healthy but do contain a higher unsaturated fat content.

- **Fat:** Unsaturated fats are the optimum with Monounsaturated, (Olive oil, almonds, etc) and Polyunsaturated (Omega 3, 6 and 9). Small amounts of saturated fats obtained from natural foods such as meat, dairy, and eggs are also healthy. It is extremely important to avoid other saturated fats (baked goods, lard, processed foods) and trans fat/esterified fats.

- **Processed foods**: Try to avoid completely, or as a minimum become a label reader and choose healthy combinations.
- **Restaurant eating:** It is easy to overeat and overdo on fat and sodium intake when eating out. Order healthy combinations and substitute vegetables for potatoes or rice. Consider ordering off the appetizer menu or plan on taking half of your meal home for leftovers on another day. Many restaurants have a pre planned lighter menu so take advantage of this.
- **Fast foods:** Rarely a great choice but Subway has done an excellent job at maximizing the nutritional value of many parts of their menu. Remember not all offerings at Subway are healthy.
- **Planning:** At the beginning of each week set out your meal schedule and shop appropriately. Pre-make your snacks the evening before to insure a healthy choice. One of my favorite snack combinations is celery, baby carrots, and grape tomatoes. Add a small smear of peanut butter onto the celery as this will promote satiety (full feeling) and help prevent overeating.

Quick tip

Nutrition is the key to weight loss with smaller, more frequent meals/snacks with healthy carbohydrates, lean protein, and primarily unsaturated fats.

Other popular diets:

- **ABS Diet:** My personal favorite. This diet is based on intelligent eating with 6 small meals per day and a regular exercise regiment. It was developed by the Men's Health Magazine Editor and the correct foods are emphasized with the acronym ABS DIET POWER.

- ✓ **A:** Almonds
- ✓ **B:** Beans and Legumes
- ✓ **S:** Spinach and other green vegetables
- ✓ **D:** Dairy- fat free or low fat milk, yogurt, and cheese
- ✓ **I:** Instant oatmeal- unsweetened and unflavored
- ✓ **E:** Eggs
- ✓ **T:** Turkey and other lean meat
- ✓ **P:** Peanut butter
- ✓ **O:** Olive oil
- ✓ **W:** Whole grain breads and cereal
- ✓ **E:** Extra protein with whey protein
- ✓ **R:** Raspberries and other berries

- **Adkins diet:** The Adkins diet clearly is an effective weight loss program but with a potential price. The intake of protein and fat without carbohydrates creates and process in the body called ketosis where your body burns fat but also muscle to maintain normal body function. This ketosis stresses the kidneys, heart, lungs, and other organs. When the Adkins diet is used long term it may result in permanent damage to various body organs. If you are planning on using this diet anyway I would suggest a short term Atkins diet to start the weight loss (for 1-2 months) and then convert to a healthy lifestyle. This diet is **NOT** a long term answer to weight loss.

- **South Beach diet:** Low carbohydrate diet with intelligent lean protein and appropriate fat intake. After the initial no carb phase this diet adds in the "good" carbohydrates. Certainly a much better plan overall and initially appeared to be an excellent diet. The major problems with this diet is that it does not emphasis exercise and it is now very clear that after the initial weight loss with a low/very low carb diet you will commonly gain the weight back and frequently overshoot your original weight. The key in carbohydrate intake is to concentrate on eating the correct carbs.

- **NutriSystem:** Based on the glycemic index with prepackaged foods that lay out the diet for you. You add the fresh fruit products. Overall an excellent diet although the food is mediocre tasting.

- **Weight Watchers:** Excellent program generally based on the glycemic index. There is no question that spending $$ improves the weight loss success by increasing motivation.

- **Sonoma Diet:** Considered the Western Hemisphere Mediterranean Diet. The Mediterranean region follows a healthy diet with unsaturated fats, healthy vegetables and fruits, and correct combinations of food. This is simply an intelligent, reasonable diet.

- **Other fad diets:** Multiple poor fad diets to include: **Cabbage soup diet** (primarily eating cabbage soup with a very low calorie diet), **Bite diet** (only a defined number of bites per day but does not restrict what foods you can eat), **Cardio free diet** (premise that exercise is bad for you), **Coconut diet** (use coconut oil to increase metabolism), **Grapefruit diet** (eating grapefruit before meals to increase metabolism), **Blood type diet** (different blood types eat different foods), **Fat flush diet** (detoxify the liver), and the **Tart diet** (juicing with maple syrup, lemon juice, water, and cayenne pepper). All of these diets are very poor and frequently became popular due to celebrity participation.

Quick tip

There are many excellent diets available. If you feel the need for a published structured diet I would suggest the ABS Diet. NutriSystem, Weight Watchers, and the Sonoma diet are also very reasonable. When you are in a plateau phase, consider changing briefly to a different diet to try and stimulate your weight loss once again. Also watch your food intake very carefully and continue to use a food diary. Remember to quickly switch back to an intelligent diet.

Exercise keys

- **Clearance:** Insure appropriate medical clearance from your primary physician.
- **Warm up/Stretch/Cool down:** Prevent injury with the correct warm up time and stretching prior to starting your exercise session. Don't forget to cool down which is essentially the warm up and stretching phase at the end.
- **Aerobic: Minimum is 3-4 times per week** with at least 30 minutes per day. Aerobic exercise sessions are additive over the course of the day so three 15 minutes sessions spread over the day count the same as one 45 minute

session. Insure that each short session has maximum effort during the entire time. The optimum weight loss is obtained with **6 days of aerobic exercise per week** with a minimum of 30 minutes per day. Options include running, power walking, biking, stationary biking (upright or semi-recumbent), elliptical, treadmill, cross country skiing, snowshoeing, and swimming.

- **Anaerobic:** Weight lifting 2-4 times per week is crucial. Initially during the session the exercise will be anaerobic (without oxygen), but after completion of the session your body will change to an aerobic (with oxygen) metabolism for the next 8-12 hours which is extremely beneficial. Low grade fat burning will occur during this extended aerobic recovery time. Also by toning your muscles you will inherently burn more calories on a daily basis as muscles requires constant energy to maintain their structure. Finally you will feel and look better with toned muscles.

- **Combined:** If the plan is to do aerobic and anaerobic exercise on the same day, the best recommendation is to proceed with the aerobic session first followed by the anaerobic portion of your work out. Scattered recent data suggest that the reverse is true and the anaerobic should be done first. There are occasional people where this reverse works better. Remember to warm up if you do the weight lifting first. This will help prevent injury.

Quick tip

Exercise is the second building block in a successful weight loss program. Regular exercise sessions during the week will promote a healthy lifestyle. When you are having a "bad" week insure that you push yourself to exercise 1-2 times that week so your training does not regress.

Pharmaceutical weight loss

- **Background:** Pharmacological weight loss is only an adjunctive therapy to nutrition and exercise. There are minimal results with the medications without following a full weight loss program with particular emphasis to nutrition and exercise. When used appropriately the medications can add an additional weight loss of 10-30 lbs. It is imperative to continue the lifestyle changes after the medical treatment is complete or you will quickly regain the weight. These medications should clearly be monitored by a physician trained in weight loss therapy.

- **Breast feeding/Pregnant/Children/Older adults:** The safety data in these groups are sketchy and these medications should not be used. Treatment age range should be 18 to 65. When storing these medications always keep them out of reach of children.
- **Other medications:** Interactions with other medications are common. Be sure to make sure your treating physician is well aware of all medications that you are on: this includes over the counter medications, herbal supplements, super nutritional supplements, illicit drugs, etc. Common medications which may result in interactions include: Amantadine (Symmetrel), Amphetamines, Caffeine, Chlorphedianol (Ulone), Cocaine, Asthma medications, Cold/Sinus/Hayfever medications, Methylphenidate (Ritalin), Nabilone (Cesamet), Pemoline (Cylert), other appetite suppressants, Selective serotonin reuptake inhibitors (Celexa, Prozac, Luvox, Paxil, Zoloft), Monoamine oxidase (MAO) inhibitors (Marplan, Nardil, Matulane, Eldepryl, Parnate), and Tricyclic antidepressants (Elavil, Asendin, Anafranil, Pertofrane, Sinequan, Tofranil, Aventyl, Vivactil, Surmontil). The interactions can be severe and include hypertensive crisis, irregular heartbeat, irritability, nervousness, tremulousness, depression, and mental illness.
- **Other medical problems:** Be sure you have updated your physician on all of your medical problems, even the problems that are completely controlled. Treatment problems can occur with alcohol abuse, drug abuse, diabetes, seizure disorder or epilepsy, mental illness, family history of mental illness, glaucoma, heart or blood vessel disease, hypertension (high blood pressure), hyperthyroidism (overactive thyroid gland), and renal or kidney disease.
- **Cholelithiasis:** Gallstones may form in patients undergoing weight loss, and particularly in patients who have frequent large variations in their weight.
- **Addiction:** These medications do have the potential for addiction, particularly in people with an addictive personality.
- **Missed doses:** If you miss a dose simply skip the dose. Do **NOT** double the dose at the next scheduled time.

- **Common prescription medications:** 1-5 are sympathomimetic appetite suppressants: 6 inhibits fat absorption
    1. **Phentermine: Adipex, Anoxine-AM, Fastin, Ionamin, Obephen, Obermine, Obestin-30, Phantrol.** These medications work by suppressing your appetite. They may be habit forming and should only be used for a maximum of 3-6 weeks. Common side effects include dry mouth, diarrhea and/or constipation, vomiting, increased blood pressure, heart palpitations, restlessness, tremulousness, dizziness, insomnia, shortness of breath, chest pain, and ankle swelling.
    2. **Sibutramine: Meridia.** The medication works by suppressing your appetite. It may be habit forming and should only be used for 3-6 weeks. Generally side effects are fairly rare but include headache, constipation, abdominal pain, insomnia, back pain, dry mouth, nervousness, tremulousness, runny nose, mood changes, heart irregularity, ankle swelling, vomiting, excessive sweating, confusion, loss of consciousness, coordination problems, seizures, chest pain, rash/hives, dilated pupils, and anxiety.
    3. **Diethylpropion: Tenuate, Tenuate Dospon.** These also work by suppressing your appetite. All of the medications may be habit forming and their use should be kept to 3-6 weeks, maximum. Side effects are not common but include dry mouth, restlessness, anxiety, depression, abdominal pain, vomiting, heart palpitations, chest pain, difficulty breathing, skin rash, fever, sore throat, painful urination, ankle swelling, and increased urination.
    4. **Phendimetrazine:** Extended release capsules that can be taken once a day. Potentially this medication is habit forming and should be used short term such as 3-6 weeks. Side effect profile is the same as Phentermine.
    5. **Benzphetamine:** Appetite suppressant which may be habit forming. As with the other sympathomimetic appetite suppressants it should be used short term, such as 3-6 weeks. Side effect profiles the same as Phentermine.
    6. **Orlistat: Xenical (prescription), Alli (over the counter):** Work in the intestines by inhibiting fat absorption. These medications may be used longer term as the side effects are fairly minimal. Diarrhea with oily stools is common due to blockage of fat absorption by the medication and therefore excess fat excretion. The oily stools can

be minimized by carefully controlling your fat intake. These medicines commonly cause fat soluble vitamin malabsorption and it is very important to take one multiple vitamin daily with the optimum time just before bed. This will insure adequate absorption of the vitamin supplement as the Orlistat or Alli should be out of your system by that time.

- **Common over the counter/herbal medications:** This is an area which requires careful examination of these products as they will commonly make broad claims of success with minimal scientific documentation. Many of the supplements will contain additives which are not listed on the label. These additives may be potentially medically dangerous.

Quick tip

Generally these supplements have little scientific proof of efficacy. Be very careful with supplements which contain Hoodia as this herb may be dangerous. Chromium picolinate may have some benefit with fat loss, and after the fat loss has been achieved CLA (Conjugated linoleic acid) may help keep the fat off. Both appear to have minimal side effects. The stacking regiment also appears to be safe overall. Alli does not appear to have any major downside if you take appropriate vitamin supplementation.

** Indicate my personal recommendations

1. ****Conjugated linoleic acid (CLA):** Works best when taken daily to maintain the weight and fat loss already achieved and is reasonable to add to your regimen as you are reaching your goal

weight. It does not appear to help with fat/weight loss by itself. There is some acceptably good data to back this.

2. **Chromium Picolinate:** Daily intake may help with fat and weight loss and is very reasonable to take on a daily basis. The data is very conflicting but chromium picolinate does not appear to have any significant down side.

3. **Stacking regiment:** To decrease fat and weight: Arginine (Nitrous oxide (NO) stimulator), glutamine, and GABA. NO stimulation scientifically makes sense and glutamine is an excellent nutritional supplement. There does not appear to be a major down side to this regiment.

4. **Green Tea:** Excellent antioxidant effect with some data suggesting a fat burning component. No significant down side and can be used on a daily basis and is a personal favorite of mine. My suggestion is one cup of hot green tea daily.

5. **Wu- Yi Tea:** Twice a day intake of a tea grown in China. The program also states that exercise and nutrition are equally important. The tea is taken twice a day and reportedly prevents food cravings, increases metabolism, and is high in polymerized polyphenols which activate enzymes to help dissolve triglycerides.

6. **Orovo:** Contains the 10 highly concentrated extracts from the 10 foods which were recommended by Dermatologist Dr. Perricone. These foods were designed to decrease wrinkles but were then noted to help with weight loss. The current Orovo product includes the extracts from the 10 super foods and 4 additional antioxidants.

7. **Nuphedragen:** Some degree of controversy surrounds this compound as it contains phenylethylamine (found in chocolate which stimulates mood improvement) and synpehrine HCL (a chemical cousin to ephedra). Be very careful with this product, particularly if there is any cardiac history.

8. **Noxycut:** Designed for men over 21 years of age. Contains fat burners and testosterone stimulation to increase muscle mass. Although you gain muscle mass and lose fat you may lose less weight (in pounds) as muscle weighs more than fat. There is significant question as to the accuracy of the claims.

9. **7-DFB:** Contains 34 natural detoxifying ingredients which are reported to flush fat out of the body. The program is combined with

a Smart Carb diet. Detoxifying agents are questionable especially with "34" in the formula.

10. **Hydroxycut:** Metabolism booster which is very popular and well known. Initially excellent results were related to the ephedrine content but it is now ephedrine free. The company states that it has maintained its fat burning potential. Hydroxycut is used by many bodybuilders with apparently some success.

11. **Xenedrine EFX:** Also a metabolism booster which now is ephedrine free. Contains other herbal supplements to help burn fat.

12. **Curvatrim:** Designed for women to help weight loss, breast enhancement, acne, and sexual vigor. Too many good claims for one pill but would be great if it were true.

13. ****Alli:** Blocks fat absorption from the intestine. Commonly causes diarrhea, oily stools, and fat soluble vitamin malabsorption. I don't see any major down side to this medication as long as you take appropriate vitamin supplements.

14. **Chitosol, Fat absorber TDSL:** Contain chitosan, a shellfish extract that blocks fat absorption from the intestines. It also causes diarrhea, oily stools, and fat soluble vitamin malabsorption. Is also associated with allergic reactions.

15. **EZ Trim, Trimspa, CarbSpa:** Contain Chromium picolinate or Vanadium which are used to block carbohydrate absorption and metabolism. Why not save the money and buy a reputable less expensive brand of Chromium picolinate?

16. **CortiDiet, CortiSlim, CortiSol, Relacare:** All reportedly decrease cortisol levels and therefore decrease excess belly fat. Very little suggestion that these work.

17. **Long list:** Many weight loss and fat burning pills are available over the counter without a prescription. As an individual you may elect to try these but remember there is no acceptable scientific data to support most of the compounds.

Quick tip

Dietary supplements (prescribed or over the counter) play only a small role in weight loss and a healthy lifestyle. The key is still lifestyle changes with emphasis to nutrition and exercise. This will accomplish your long term goal of wellness.

Part V

Integrative Medicine

Preventative Medicine

Preventative medicine is the practice of screening for asymptomatic diseases before clinical problems develop or the teaching of lifestyle changes which may improve the person's overall health thereby preventing disease and accident occurrence. Many recommendations are proposed but not all proposals are appropriate. The United States Preventive Services Task Force (USPSTF) is an independent panel of expects who review the current data and come to a consensus based on scientific data as to which screening recommendations are the most reasonable. International recommendations may vary from country to country based on the opinions of the data. The following outline contain screening recommendations and point out the controversial areas. Not all of the following recommendations follow the USPSTF recommendations as many incorporate suggestions/recommendations from other sources.

Screening

- **Physical examinations:** Regular visits to your physician should be based on your overall health. Generally regular adult examinations are considered every 5 years starting at age 25, but are done with more frequent intervals if there are any active medical problems. Blood pressure and other screening can be done without a full physical examination. Routine physicals on a more frequent basis have not been shown to be beneficial in preventing disease but I don't understand the down side to intermittent examinations. I question if this data is driven by insurance companies to save $$. Therefore my suggestion is a routine physical examination every 5 years starting at 25 and every 1-3 years starting at age 50.
- **Height and Weight:** Periodically these should be checked and should clearly be done with each physical exam. BMI (Body Mass Index) greater than 30 in general are considered obese and should work particularly hard on weight management. Athletic people with a higher muscle mass will have a higher BMI (even over 30) but may not be considered obese due to the fact that muscle weighs more than fat and the BMI calculations do not account for this. In this situation a measurement of Body Fat is necessary.

- **Blood pressure:** It is important to check every a blood pressure every 2 years, or more frequently if there are any borderline readings or a trend towards a higher blood pressure. Generally 120/80 is considered normal. One elevated blood pressure does not indicate the presence of hypertension and serial BP checks are used to make this diagnosis. The top number is called the systolic BP and the bottom number is the diastolic. The systolic BP has a greater tendency to vary and may go up to some degree with stress and anxiety whereas the diastolic number does not vary like this. If you are doing home or store BP checks, a general rule of thumb is that BP greater than 140/90 is concerning. Maintain a BP log and discuss this with your physician. Hypertension (High Blood Pressure) is a silent disease and is commonly without symptoms. Prolonged hypertension increases your risk of strokes, heart disease, and kidney disease.
- **Diabetes Mellitus:** Routine screening is debatable but should start at age 45 in most people. Earlier and more frequent screenings should occur in people with a family history of diabetes or if you have hypertension and/or hyperlipidemia (high cholesterol). Personally I would recommend screening once in the 20's and once in the 30's with additional screenings at any time routine blood work is done. A serum glucose (sugar) check is very inexpensive.
- **Lipid screen:** Total cholesterol and HDL cholesterol (or better yet full lipid panel with total cholesterol, LDL cholesterol, HDL cholesterol, and triglycerides) in men over 35 and women over 45. An additional screening earlier at age 20 to 25 is also very reasonable and is suggested by many sources but not recommended by the USPSTF. People with other heart risk factors such as diabetes and hypertension should be screened every 5 years. The data is excellent that controlling cholesterol decreases the prevalence of heart disease and strokes. The data on triglycerides currently does not correlate with heart disease, but triglyceride levels over 600 increases the risk of pancreatitis.
- **Colorectal cancer:** Colonoscopy at age 50 and repeat every 5-10 years. Follow up interval would change if there are adenomatous polyps removed during the initial colonoscopy. Adenomatous polyps have the potential to degenerate into colon cancer over the years. Once a colon starts to form these polyps they may continue to intermittently form over time. If there is a family history of colon cancer (first degree relative under the age of 60 or two first degree relatives at any age) then the initial

colonoscopy should be at age 40, or 10 years before the earliest onset of colon cancer in the family. Someday CT Colography/Virtual colonoscopy and Stool DNA testing may play a role, but the data is still questionable.

- **Mammogram:** Every 1-2 years for women over the age of 40 and yearly after age 50. The data on self breast exam is debatable but each woman should still perform this monthly with a physician breast exam with each GYN physical (every 2-3 years). Self breast examination is free and many women will find small changes in their breasts.

- **Pap test:** For cervical cancer. Should be done every 3 years from the age of sexual activity until age 65 but the interval should be decreased if there is an abnormal Pap smear. Pap smears can be discontinued after a hysterectomy for benign disease.

- **Chlamydia screen:** Sexually active women under 25 or high risk women at any age should be screened for chlamydia.

- **Bone density:** Women over 65 and earlier for anyone with higher risk. This would include chronic steroid use, family history of osteoporosis, personal history of bone fracture, prostate cancer treatment, early menopause, hypogonadism, prolonged hyperthyroidism, celiac sprue, and anorexia nervosa/other eating disorders. Personally I believe a screening at age 50 is a very reasonable baseline as osteoporosis treatment is more effective when started early.

- **Thyroid screening:** Particularly important for the diagnosis of hypothyroidism (under functioning thyroid). It is also reasonable in post partum (after delivery) and post menopausal women, elderly, patients with diabetes, and patients with Down's syndrome.

- **AAA screening:** For abdominal aortic aneurysm. Recommended in men age 65-75 who have smoked at any time in their life. AAA rupture is usually fatal therefore early detection is imperative.

- **Depression:** During routine physician's visit a simple screening for major depression is appropriate. Questions include: "Over the past 2 weeks have you felt down, depressed, or hopeless?" and "Over the past 2 weeks have you felt little or no interest or pleasure in doing things?" A more extensive evaluation would be indicated in anyone who may be depressed as control of depression promotes wellness.

- **Alcohol Abuse/Misuse:** Screening involves simply asking "how many alcoholic drinks do you have daily." Over 2 drinks per day (or many times per week) or binge drinking may result in significant problems including end stage liver disease. Small amounts of alcohol may actually have a protective effect on the heart, but this data should not be used as an excuse to drink excessively. It is extremely important to screen pregnant women and emphasis the detrimental effects of alcohol on the fetus. Pregnant women should not drink any alcohol.

- **Vision screening:** Start at age 65 or earlier if there are any questions about their visual acuity. The elderly commonly deny problems and must be specifically screened. Early detection of vision or hearing problems may help the elderly maintain their independence which is extremely important. Simple vision screening charts are used with referral to an Optometrist and Ophthalmologist if there are any abnormalities.

- **Hearing screening:** Start at age 65 or earlier if there are any questions about their hearing. The elderly commonly deny problems and must be specifically screened. A portable audioscope or screening oral questionnaire may be used.

- **Prostate cancer:** The data on screening is controversial and studies are ongoing. The USPSTF does not have any current screening recommendations but in my opinion a prostate exam during the normal physical exam is important and a PSA (blood test) at age 50-55 is reasonable.

- **Ovarian cancer:** Screening with Vaginal Ultrasound and/or CA-125 (tumor marker) does detect a small percentage of ovarian cancer earlier but is not recommended for screening as there is a high number of false positives which require evaluation. This results in an unacceptably high number of negative invasive procedures which result in morbidity (complications). This clearly outweighs the benefits of screening. Routine pelvic examination and Pap smear every 3 years should be done.

- **Heart disease:** Routine screening generally is not recommended. Consider exceptions in people with a sedentary lifestyle who are about to embark on an exercise program, people with a strong family history of cardiac disease, and people with other cardiac risk factor problems such as diabetes, hypertension, or hyperlipidemia. Screening procedures include any combination of EKG, Exercise or Chemical Stress Test, and electron beam CT. Certainly high risk patients will benefit from control of their underlying medical problems, and obviously should not be smoking.

- **Carotid artery stenosis screening:** Neither physical exam or ultrasound screening has been shown to be beneficial. Smoking predisposes to peripheral vascular disease and is a major health and wellness risk.

Smoking should be avoided by all but high risk atherosclerotic disease patients clearly should not be smoking.

- **Tuberculosis screening:** TB tests should be done only in high risk groups which include health care workers, immigrants from endemic regions, migrant workers, homeless patients, alcoholics, and people who have an exposure history to TB.
- **Skin cancer screening:** Total body skin examination has not been shown to be beneficial but is essentially free and without risks. In my opinion this should be done with each regular physical examination and each person should be taught to do self examinations. Place an emphasis on any change in color or character of a mole as this should be reported to their primary physician ASAP. These changes may suggest the onset of a melanoma, the most aggressive form of skin cancer.
- **Bladder, Ovary, Lung, Mouth, and Pancreas screening:** Overall screening for these problems is ineffective in multiple studies. Despite this, oral visual and palpation examination during routine physical exam or by a dentist during routine cleaning is very reasonable in my opinion. Lung cancer can be screened with chest XR with minimal risks or costs and should be considered in high risk patients such as smokers and prior exposure to carcinogens such as miners and asbestos workers.
- **My take:** Make sure your primary care physician is providing the appropriate medical screening. You must be an advocate for your health and wellness.

Diet and exercise

- **Nutrition recommendations:** Multiple small food servings daily, appropriate carbohydrates with whole wheat/fruits/vegetables, lean protein, and emphasize unsaturated fat.
- **Exercise recommendations:** Regular physical activity 3-4 times per week with 30 minutes or greater per session (remember vigorous sessions can be additive over the course of the day). This may be a formal exercise routine or participation in an athletic event that has a significant aerobic component.
- **My take:** Eat correctly and exercise regularly.

Substance abuse

- **Smoking and tobacco cessation:** This will decrease a person's risk of lung disease (COPD), lung carcinoma, heart disease, strokes, peripheral vascular disease, pancreatic carcinoma, esophageal cancer, colon cancer, bladder cancer, and multiple other significant medical problems. This may be the single most important lifestyle change a person can do to improve on wellness.
- **Alcohol cessation:** It is extremely important to discontinue regular excessive alcohol intake (greater the 2 drinks per day several times per week) or frequent binge drinking. This decreases the incidence of liver disease, chronic pancreatitis, CNS (brain) related damage, heart damage, and potentially liver/pancreatic carcinoma.
- **Illicit drug use:** There is no circumstance where illicit drug use would medically benefit the person. Any consideration of marijuana use for chronic nausea should involve medical formulations of marijuana and be supervised by a physician.
- **My take:** Tobacco, excessive alcohol, and illicit drugs are obstacles to health and wellness. Eliminate these problems.

Injury prevention

- **Safety belts:** Lap and shoulder belts should be used in both front and back seats for all passengers in a car and if possible in a bus and other forms of transportation. Try and purchase a car/SUV/truck with front and side air bags. When used appropriately, seat belts and air bags decrease morbidity and mortality associated with accidents.
- **Helmets:** Head protection is important at all times for motorcycle, bicycle, and ATV use and clearly decrease the incidence and severity of head injuries.
- **Firearms:** Safe storage of firearms to prevent unintended use decreases the accidental discharge rate. If small children are in the house at any time it is very important to have a locking system. Keep the ammunition separate for extra protection. Accidental firearm discharge is a far too common cause of childhood death.
- **Smoke and CO (Carbon monoxide) detectors:** Should cover the entire house. It is important to change the batteries yearly or use electrical power with battery backup (change to backup batteries yearly).

Adequate warning during a house fire could save your life. CO2 is an odorless gas which can build up and result in death.

- **Alcohol:** It is important to not drink alcohol while driving (car, motorcycle, scooter, ATV, bicycle, bus, etc), boating, wave runner, jet ski, or swimming. Alcohol intake increases the injury and death rate for the driver, passengers, pedestrians, and other vehicle occupants. There are also major legal ramifications with alcohol intake in these situations and prison time is not conducive to wellness.
- **Sun exposure:** All exposed skin areas need appropriate protection with sun screen or clothing. SFP 15 to 45 will provide protection to exposed areas such as the face, ears, arms, legs, etc. Don't forget to cover your lips with lip balm with at least SPF 15 and men who are bald don't forget the top of your head. Cloudy days can still result in significant ultraviolet light exposure therefore sun screen is still necessary on those days. Sun screen can prevent severe sun burns and potentially decrease the incidence of skin cancer. Most commercial sunscreens protect against the UVB rays but UVA rays can also cause sunburn and skin cancer. Try to find a sunscreen which protects against UVB and UVA rays. Remember to protect your cornea (eyes) with polarized sun glasses as this will prevent corneal burns. These burns are particularly severe when in a snowy area as the light reflects off the snow and causes a double UV ray exposure.
- **My take:** Protect yourself, these are all important recommendations.

Dental health

- **Dental visits:** Regular dental examinations and cleaning will protect your oral region and promote wellness. The minimum is yearly or as directed by your dentist.
- **Daily cleaning:** Brush with fluoride toothpaste and floss daily to twice a day. Don't forget to brush your tongue. There is some data suggesting that using a Listerine type mouthwash helps to decrease plaque, tarter, and bacterial problems.
- **My take:** Protect your teeth. You only get one set during adulthood and poor dental hygiene may predispose to multiple different infections.

Sexual behavior

- **Contraception:** To prevent unintended pregnancy employ effective contraceptive methods.
- **STD education:** Careful with high risk sexual behavior and use condoms.
- **STD screening:** Important in people with high risk behavior to be screened. This includes promiscuity, unprotected sexual intercourse, prostitute exposure, anal intercourse, and history of prior STD. Periodic HIV and Syphilis serology should be performed and a strong consideration should be given to hepatitis screening for both Chronic Hepatitis B (clearly sexually transmitted) and Hepatitis C (transmitted sexually to a very small degree). Sexual active women under 25 should have Chlamydia and HPV screening. Consider HPV vaccine in young females before the onset of sexual intercourse.
- **My take:** Condoms should be used whenever the situation is not a long term monogamous relationship and STD screening is important.

Chemoprevention: daily supplement intake to promote wellness

- **Multiple vitamin:** All adults should take a multivitamin with minerals daily. For pregnant woman, a daily prenatal vitamin which should contain folic acid. Generally the average diet has multiple nutritional deficiencies and a daily multivitamin will help overcome these deficiencies.
- **Calcium:** Daily supplementation with calcium and Vitamin D in all peri and post menopausal women is very important. Supplementation should also be done with any person on chronic steroids, a family history of osteoporosis, personal history of unexplained bone fracture, and patients on prostate cancer treatment (hormonal therapy). People in northern states (above a line from Philadelphia to San Francisco) who have suboptimal intake of Vitamin D fortified foods should also take supplements. Adequate calcium and Vitamin D intake helps protect against bone disease.
- **Low dose Aspirin:** All men over 40 and all women over 50 should take a safety (enteric) coated 81mg aspirin daily. This may be considered earlier if there is a family history of heart disease starting at an early age. Low dose aspirin helps protect against heart attacks and strokes.
- **Omega-3:** Daily intake with a minimum of 600mg of EPA and DHA Omega 3. In general, our intake of Omega 3 is suboptimal and the dietary ratio of Omega 6 to Omega 3 is incorrect which results in

increased generalized inflammation in the body. This ratio can be corrected with supplementation. Adequate Omega 6 to 3 ratio decreases heart disease and inflammation.

- **Super B complex:** B vitamins can be difficult to obtain in a normal diet. Extra Vitamin B intake is safe as this is a water soluble vitamin and any excess will be excreted through the kidneys. Daily supplementation is very helpful in preventing the multiple problems associated with B deficiencies.
- **Fiber:** Daily fiber intake should be 20-30 grams. This is commonly difficult to obtain and a supplementation of 3-5 grams per day is healthy. Adequate fiber promotes a healthy digestive system, decreases cholesterol, and improves glucose control.
- **Probiotics:** Daily supplementation of "good" intestinal bacteria promotes a healthy GI tract. 2-30 billion per day is a reasonable recommendation. Find a supplement with this dose so only one capsule per day is necessary. Refrigerated, liquid probiotics do not supply any additional benefit over the capsule form but are more expensive.
- **My take:** These are all important supplements.

Vaccinations

Influenza: The flu requires a yearly vaccine as the strains of will vary from year to year and the vaccine is designed to protect against the highest probability strains for that year. People with a documented fever, prior severe reaction to the vaccine, or an egg allergy should not receive the vaccine. The main vaccine is an inactivated virus but an intranasal live vaccine is available for people aged 5 to 49. The live vaccine should not be given to people who are pregnant or immunocompromised.

- **Routine:** Yearly for all people equal to or over 65.
- **High risk situations:** Yearly for people with chronic heart disease, chronic lung disease (COPD and asthma), diabetes, chronic renal disease, immunosuppression, pregnant women whose last 2 trimesters coincide

with the flu season, or hemoglobinopathies. Consider in college students, nursing home residents, workers exposed to multiple different groups of people on a daily basis, and prisoners.

- **High risk occupations:** Yearly for health care workers including long term care facilities, and day care workers.
- **My take:** A flu vaccine yearly for all adults is reasonable and important. The risks of the vaccine are low and the benefits are potentially enormous.

Pneumococcal: The PPV-23 protects against 23 antigen types of streptococcal pneumonia with 60% efficaciousness in preventing bacteremia. Bacteremia is the main cause of morbidity in pneumococcal disease. Immunity wanes after 5 years therefore a booster is necessary.

- **Routine:** At age 65 and every 5 years after this.
- **Risk factors:** Every 5 years in people with chronic heart disease, chronic lung disease, diabetes, chronic liver disease (particularly alcoholic liver disease), chronic renal disease, immunosuppression, status post splenectomy, functional asplenia, and people on chemotherapy.
- **My take:** The recommendations are appropriate.

Hepatitis A: One time vaccination with two doses over 6 months. There is also a Hepatitis A vaccine that contains an immunoglobulin. This vaccine is used in people traveling to endemic areas who require rapid immunity. It is very reasonable for all people to obtain the vaccine as there have been sporadic outbreaks of Hepatitis A in the US. Raw shellfish such as oysters and clams may contain Hepatitis A but food handlers may also transmit the virus while they are preparing the food. There is a combined Hepatitis A and B vaccine for people who have never had either vaccine.

- **Occupational:** Travelers, food handlers, and plumbers are mandatory from a health standpoint. The vaccine should be strongly considered in health care workers and day care workers.
- **High risk:** Chronic liver disease, men who have sex with men, and illicit drug users should all be vaccinated.
- **My take:** All people should be vaccinated against Hepatitis A.

Hepatitis B: Series of three injections over 6 months given at 0, 1, and 6 months. Currently a booster is not recommended if there is an adequate response to the initial vaccine and the immunity is maintained (check a serum HBsAb- if positive the patient is immune).

- **Routine:** Many states now require all young adults to have the vaccine before entering 7th grade. This is an excellent recommendation.
- **High risks:** Healthcare workers, public safety workers, IV Illicit drug users, promiscuous people, men who have sex with men, and recently acquired STD.
- **Serological response:** Check HBsAb to insure adequate response. Check for immunity with serology every 10 years and if the HBsAb is negative a single booster dose is appropriate.
- **My take:** All people should be vaccinated against Hepatitis B.

Tetanus/Diphtheria (Td): Initial is a series of 3 injections at 0, 1, and 6 months to prevent "lock jaw." All people should maintain their immunity to tetanus and diphtheria with a booster every 10 years.

- **Routine:** Complete primary (3 dose series) and then a booster every 10 years. All new residents of the US should receive the initial series (3 injections) if it was never given in the past.
- **Puncture wound:** Additional dose when any potentially dirty laceration or puncture wound occurs.
- **My take:** Keep your Td vaccine up to date.

MMR: To prevent mumps, measles, and rubella. Recommended and generally required during childhood.

- **Prior infection:** Most people born before 1956 were infected during childhood. Screen and vaccinate anyone born after 1956 that does not have proof of immunity.
- **High risk:** Health care workers, international travelers, and day care workers. Prior to becoming pregnant women should be screened for immunity to rubella and given the MMR if the rubella serology is negative. The vaccine is contraindicated in women who are already pregnant.

Vaccinations should also be done during an institutional outbreak in people without documented immunity.

- **Booster:** All adolescents should receive a booster due to the outbreaks in colleges.
- **My take:** The recommendations are appropriate.

Varicella: To prevent Chicken pox. The vaccine is contraindicated in pregnant women, immunocompromised, and individuals taking more than 20mg per day of steroids. Avoid close contact with immunocompromised individuals for 4 weeks after receiving the vaccine as there is a low potential for infecting this person. A rash occasionally will be a complication of the vaccine.

- **High risk:** Health care workers, family contacts of immunocompromised persons, teachers, child care providers, residents and staff in institutional settings.
- **Childbearing age:** Should be given to all nonpregnant women of childbearing age who do not have immunity. The vaccine is contraindicated to pregnant women.
- **My take:** The recommendations are appropriate.

Polio: Oral vaccine to prevent polio which can cause severe neurological damage.

- **Routine:** Generally not indicated for adults but consider vaccination if primary series was never completed.
- **My take:** Complete the vaccine if it was never done.

Shingles vaccine (Herpes Zoster): New vaccine that should be given even if you have had Shingles in the past.

- **Routine:** Indicated for all adults over the age of 60.
- **My take:** The recommendations are appropriate.

Meningococcal:

- **Routine:** Not recommended for adults who are without a high risk situation. Is now recommended for adolescents particularly if going to college and staying in the dormitory.
- **High risk:** Travelers (particularly to sub-Sahara Africa), and college dormitory residents. Immunization also suggested during local outbreaks.
- **My take:** The recommendations are appropriate.

Herbal and Super Nutritional Supplements

Herbal and Super Nutritional Supplement Rules

Quick tip:

Herbal medications can be extremely beneficial, but all users need to keep several thoughts in mind before starting these compounds. See the list below.

- Remember these compounds are not regulated by the FDA (Food and Drug Administration) and therefore scientific proof is not needed to make any specific claim of success.
- These compounds are medications. Be sure to discuss their use with your physician and before surgery provide your medical team with a list of your supplements. This includes your primary care physician, any consulting physician, the surgeon, and particularly the anesthesiologist/nurse anesthetist.
- Include these compounds on your medication list and carry this list with you in your wallet at all times.
- Be sure to research any known drug interactions before starting the medication, including interactions with your present medications.
- Don't overdo it. More is not necessarily better so follow the dosage recommendation as listed on the package, or use a dose published in a respected book.

- Careful with what you buy. Excellent references are obtained from the USP Seal (US Pharmacopeia's), CL Seal (ConsumerLab.com), Good Housekeeping Seal, and the NSF International Seal. These seals will insure that the pill you are taking contains the compounds listed on the label as these are independent organizations which monitor nutritional supplements. This certification does not insure that the supplement is medically safe for you, so research drug interactions, etc. before starting the supplement.

Best choices for Herbal and Super Nutritional Supplements

Ratings

- ✓ ***** **Best of the best**
- ✓ **** **Very good**
- ✓ *** **Good**
- ✓ ** **Use with some caution**
- ✓ * **Avoid**

Omega 3 Fatty Acids/Fish Oils

- Excellent choice to **lower Triglycerides, raise HDL and to some degree lower total Cholesterol and lower LDL**. In higher doses it works particularly well in decreasing the triglyceride level.
- Enteric coated preparations have been used in Crohn's disease.
- Also has anti-inflammatory properties, decrease platelet aggregation (clumping of platelets), decrease the blood pressure, and lower the risks of stoke.
- Have been reported to repair brain tissue.

- EPA (eicosapentainoic acid) and DHA (docosahexaenoic acid) are obtained from fish oil and are the best types of Omega 3. The best ratio in a supplement is 3:2 of EPA to DHA.
- ALA (alphalinoleic acid) is also useful and can be obtained from plants/nuts/seeds.
- Omega 6 is the fatty acid found in vegetable oils. When the ratio of Omega 3 to Omega 6 is out of balance the body releases chemicals that promote inflammation. Generally we eat too much Omega 6 and therefore Omega 3 supplementation is beneficial.
- Common dose: 800 to 1500 mg per day with at least 600 mg of EPA and DHA. Certain conditions may require higher doses (3 grams per day or more) but this should be done under the guidance of a physician.
- **Side effects:** Minimal overall but include fishy breath or taste in the mouth, elevated glucose levels (higher doses for longer periods of time).
- **My take: An excellent supplement which should be taken daily by everyone!!**
- **Rating: *******

Quick tip

Omega 3 fatty acids are essentially a mandatory supplement for good health and wellness unless you have sufficient intake of oily fish such as salmon, herring, tuna, and sardines.

Probiotics

- Probiotics contain one or several different bacteria which may be beneficial to your gastrointestinal track. It is unclear if one particular bacteria is the best, or if a combination of bacteria is better.
- Real Yogurt contains acidophilus but in fairly small doses.

- Excellent for gastrointestinal problems including **Irritable Bowel Syndrome, diarrhea, constipation, gas and bloating.**
- Common doses include 2-30 billion CFU (Colony Forming Units). Try to obtain a sufficient dose per tablet so you only need to take this once or maximum twice per day.
- **My take: Excellent supplement for overall gastrointestinal health. Should clearly be taken daily by anyone with chronic GI problems.**
- ➢ **Rating: *******

Quick tip

If you are not taking a probiotic regularly, then start the supplement whenever you take a course of antibiotics. Continue the probiotic during the entire course of antibiotics, then for one additional week. This will decrease the potential antibiotic related gastrointestinal side effects and for women decrease the probability of vaginal yeast infections.

Red Yeast Rice

- Similar to a Statin type drug (Crestor, Pravachol, etc) as it is a natural HMG- CoA reductase inhibitor.
- **Decreases Total Cholesterol, LDL, and to a smaller degree Triglycerides. It may also increase HDL.**
- Most beneficial in less severe cases of Hypercholesterolemia (high cholesterol).
- Common dose: 1.2 to 2.4 grams per day divided into two or three doses.
- **Side effects:** Generally well tolerated. Liver toxicity and gastrointestinal side effects with gas, bloating, indigestion have been reported.

- **My take: This is an excellent supplement option for the treatment of high cholesterol. Remember red yeast rice does not substitute for appropriate nutritional treatment with a low fat diet.**
  - **Rating: ******

> Quick tip
>
> Liver toxicity is still a risk with Red yeast rice, although small, just like patients who take a prescription statin drug (like Lipitor). Have your physician monitor your blood work (liver panel) at least every 3-6 months.

Green Tea

- Green tea, unlike black or oolong tea, is not fermented which allows the active ingredients to remain in the tea.
- High in antioxidants with polypenols and flavenoids.
- Green tea decreases cholesterol levels, and may improve heart disease by decreasing platelet aggregation and preventing clot formation in the coronary (heart) blood vessels.
- It is also recommended to help decrease myalgias and arthralgias, improve digestion, improve depression, and help with digestion.
- Antioxidant effect may decrease cancer risk.
- Has a thermogenic effect and can be used as a fat burner.
- Common dose: 270 mg per day in a pill form. 3 cups per day (750 ml) if green tea is consumed.
- Side effects: Minimal problems but insomnia and anxiety are common with caffeinated products. These effects can be modulated with the use of decaffeinated tea. Most tablet forms are decaffeinated.
- **My take: This is another potentially beneficial supplement with minimal side effects.**
- **Rating: *****

Coenzyme Q10

- Excellent antioxidant properties and helps preserve Vitamin E which is the major antioxidant of cell membranes.
- Improves oxygen conversion in muscle cells and may help in heart disease, high blood pressure, and chronic fatigue syndrome.
- Several studies suggest a benefit in patients with angina (chest pain related to a lack of blood flow to the heart muscle).
- Improves energy level
- May help in Alzheimers although the data is vague.
- Common dose: 100 mg per day with most studies using 90-150 mg per day.
- Side effects: Minimal overall, but patients with Congestive Heart Failure should not attempt to discontinue Coenzyme Q10 abruptly as this may precipitate heart failure.
- **My take: Very useful supplement particularly in people with chronic heart problems including high blood pressure and coronary insufficiency.**
- **Rating: ******

SAMe (S-adenosyl- methionine)

- Anti-inflammatory effect.
- Improves joint health and is useful in arthritis.
- Improves mood and depression by increasing dopamine in the brain. Antidepressant effects are commonly seen in one week.
- Vague data suggesting help in liver disease.
- Common dose: Osteoarthritis 800 to 1200 mg per day: Depression 1600 mg per day: Migraine 800 mg per day.
- Side effects: Occasional gastrointestinal upset but overall well tolerated.
- **My take: Very helpful supplement in people with chronic joint problems with chronic arthralgia. May be used on a daily long term basis, or may be used for short periods of time (2-6 weeks) during acute flares of arthralgias.**
- **Rating: *****

Glucosamine/Chondroitin/MSM

- Made from the skeleton of shellfish.
- May use Glucosamine alone or in combination with Chondroitin and potentially MSM.
- Anti-inflammatory effect with excellent results in mild to moderate joint disease with arthritis. Has been used exclusively for the treatment of Osteoarthritis.
- Common dose: 1000 to 2000 mg per day in divided doses.
- Side effects: Minimal but include allergic reactions, gastrointestinal upset, and glucose elevations.
- **My take: Overall a very well tolerated supplement with excellent benefits when used chronically for osteoarthritis (DJD, wear and tear) of peripheral joints such as knees, ankles, hips, etc. This supplement does not work particularly well in inflammatory diseases such as rheumatoid arthritis.**
- **Rating: ******

Quick tip

Glucosamine may be equally beneficial as Nonsteroidal anti-inflammatory medications such a Motrin, Ibuprofen, etc.

Chromium Picolinate

- Improves insulin sensitivity and may help normalize blood sugar.
- Decreases the urge to consume sugar and may be useful in diabetics.
- May be beneficial in fat burning and weight loss although the data is conflicting.
- Additional excellent source is Brewer's Yeast obtained as a byproduct of beer production. If there is not a bitter taste to the product it does not contain active Chromium.
- Common dose: 200 to 400 mcg per day.
- Side effects: Minimal in standard doses but high doses may cause hypoglycemia, kidney damage, and heart rhythm problems.

- **My take: Worth a try as a weight loss and fat mobilization supplement but would not take long term if there is no obvious benefit. Probably not of major benefit to diabetic patients.**
- **Rating: *****

Conjugated Linoleic Acid

- Best used in weight control to decrease fat formation after the desired weight is reached.
- Does not appear to assist in initial weight loss.
- May reduce the risk of various cancers including breast, prostate, colorectal, stomach, and lung.
- Common dose: 3-4 grams per day in divided doses.
- Side effects: Minimal but does increase lipid levels and increases blood glucose. Because of this should only be used short term, i.e. less than 6 months.
- **My take: Acceptable to use for 6 months after losing the fat and reaching your goal weight. If there is no obvious benefit after 1-2 months then I would discontinue the supplement.**
- **Rating: *****

Andrographis

- Common names include Chiretta, Kirata, and Chuan xin lian.
- Kan jang is an excellent prep that is combined with Siberian ginsing.
- Active ingredient is andrographolides theat have immune stimulating and anti-inflammatory properties.
- Best used for common cold type symptoms.
- If taken early decreases the duration and severity of symptoms. Appears to work extremely well.
- May help in Infectious diarrhea when combined with antibiotics.
- Common dose: 100 mg of standard extract twice a day- 500 mg to 3000 mg three times a day of the dried herb.
- Side effects: Minimal overall.
- **My take: Use this supplement short term for the common cold. Start at the earliest onset of symptoms and continue for 5-7 days.**

- Rating: ****

Ginger

- Helpful in treating nausea and vomiting and may prevent the formation of ulcers.
- Helps best with motion sickness.
- May reduce nausea and vomiting post anesthesia and with chemotherapy.
- Popular remedy for nausea and vomiting associated with pregnancy particularly with the severe form called Hyperemesis Gravidarum. Unfortunately it is unclear how safe ginger is with pregnancy .
- Tones the digestive tract and stimulates digestion.
- Has anti-inflammatory properties and inhibits platelet aggregation.
- Do not take with bleeding disorders.
- Common dose: 500-1000 mg every 4 hours.
- Side effects: Generally very safe but should not be used if you have gallstones. Ginger should not be taken within 1 week of surgery due to the antiplatelet effects, so tell your anesthesiologist and surgeon before surgery if you are taking ginger. Stop the supplement 7 days before surgery.
- **My take: There are many potential beneficial effects with ginger. It is very useful for motion sickness such as going on a cruise. Start the ginger 5 days before the cruise and continue the supplement daily until you get back. It is also worth a try in people with chronic nausea once an appropriate medical evaluation has not found any other reasons for the problem.**
- Rating: ***

Black Cohash

- Has effects that are similar to the female hormone estrogen.
- Treats perimenopausal symptoms with hot flashes, headaches, and mood disorders.

- Also treats night sweats and insomnia.
- Best if taken less than 6 months.
- Common dose: Standardized extract 20 to 40 mg twice a day. Powdered extract 250 mg three times a day.
- Side effects: Occasional gastrointestinal symptoms with abdominal pain and nausea and should not be used in pregnancy or while breast feeding. Vague reports of liver failure.
- **My take: Reasonable to take a short course to see if it is beneficial in controlling hot flashes. May also combine with soy for added benefit in the treatment of hot flashes. Do not use long term and discontinue early on if there is no benefit.**
- **Rating: *****

Soy

- Contains isoflavones which have estrogen like properties.
- Helpful for perimenopausal symptoms of hot flashes, headaches, and mood disorders.
- Additionally, an excellent source of protein, fiber, vitamins, and minerals.
- May decrease cholesterol as a side benefit.
- Common dose: 4 to 8 oz of soy milk, one serving of soy product, or 50 to 100 mg per day in tablet form.
- Side effects: Allergic reactions, constipation, and occasionally an increase in goiter size. Vague reports of higher doses of soy for longer periods of time may cause uterine hyperplasia which theoretically could increase GYN cancer risk.
- **My take: Overall very safe with a nutritious side bonus. Very reasonable to try in the treatment of perimenopausal symptoms.**
- **Rating: ******

Quick tip

Black cohash and Soy in combination are beneficial for perimenopausal symptoms. Black cohash should not used for greater than 6 months without a medication holiday.

Tumeric

- Spice used in curry.
- Active ingredient is curcumin.
- Has anti-inflammatory properties similar to COX-2 Inhibitors such as Celebrex and is useful in Degenerative Joint Disease (joint pains related to wear and tear).
- Contains an antioxidant called Quercetin.
- Has been reported to decrease colon polyp formation (John Hopkins University).
- May help in Alzheimers by decreasing plaque formation in the brain.
- Common dose: 250 to 500 mg three times a day in standardized extract capsules.
- Side effects: Minimal overall. Do not take if you have gallstones.
- **My take: Would try this supplement for arthralgias (joint pains) particularly if Glucosamine is not helpful.**
- **Rating: ******

Pycnogenol

- Overall an excellent antioxidant and may decrease the risk of cancer.
- Data suggest that it may help treat diabetes, high cholesterol, Attention Deficit Disorder, and retinopathy.
- Similar to eating vegetables and fruit.
- **My take: No major downside but it is best to obtain high quality antioxidants from fruits and vegetables.**
- **Rating: *****

Garlic

- Excellent herbal supplement with many potential beneficial effects.
- Has antibacterial, antifungal, anticancer, and enhanced immune system properties.
- Decreases blood pressure, decreases cholesterol, and decreases triglycerides.
- Clearly decreases LDL.
- Helps prevent the common cold and other infections.
- Do not take with anti-clotting medications. Tell your physicians (and anesthesiologist) before surgery that you are taking garlic.
- Common dose: Enteric coated tablets or capsules with 1.3% allin - total dose 600 to 900 mg per day divided into two or three doses. May also use 2-3 cloves a garlic per day if the odor is not a problem.
- Side effects: Minimal but may increase GERD (reflux) and may cause gas, bloating, and flatus.
- **My take: Very useful supplement for the treatment of dyslipidemia (high cholesterol and high triglycerides). Would use as an adjunctive therapy to Omega 3 and potentially Red Yeast Rice.**
- **Rating: ******

Quick tip

Active ingredient in Garlic is Allicin. This ingredient may be missing in some of the odor free tablets.

Saw Palmetto

- Helpful in treating enlarged prostate glands (Benign Prostatic Hypertrophy) potentially by reducing the amount of dihydrotestosterone (DHT) which is an active form of testosterone.
- Does not have estrogen like effects.

- Additionally saw palmetto has diuretic properties.
- Common dose: Extract in capsules 160 mg per day.
- Side effects: Overall appears very safe with minimal problems.
- **My take: Excellent choice in the treatment of BPH.**
- **Rating: ******

Quick tip

Saw palmetto does not appear to interfere with the PSA assay which is used to evaluate for prostate cancer.

Milk Thistle

- Silymarin is the active ingredient which has excellent antioxidant capabilities with flavonoids.
- Protects and detoxifies the liver.
- Has liver anti-inflammatory effects and helpful in Hepatitis C and Alcoholic Liver Disease.
- Decreases gallstone formation.
- Common dose: Standardized extract 600 mg per day.
- Side effects: None.
- **My take: Although milk thistle will not specifically treat and "cure" liver disease, the liver anti-inflammatory effects are very useful and it should be used as an adjunctive therapy particularly for Hepatitis C.**
- **Rating: ******

Glutamine

- Abundant amino acid in the body which is a nonessential aa.

- Involved in multiple metabolic processes in the body.
- Helpful in intestinal health including Irritable Bowel Syndrome and Diarrhea.
- Improves pre and post surgical health.
- Active in fat burning and muscle building for athletic performance.
- Improves immune function.
- Common dose: 2-5 grams twice a day.
- Side effects: None reported.
- **My take: Excellent supplement with no down side. Would use for infectious diarrhea, IBS, hospitalized patients with intestinal problems, and for its athletic performance properties.**
- **Rating: *****

Quick tip

Witch Hazel is an excellent salve which can be used on external hemorrhoids. Apply to the hemorrhoids after a bowel movement. This is the active ingredient in Tucks pads.

Best of the rest: Super Nutritional and Herbal Supplementation

Aloe Vera

- Has antibacterial, antifungal, and anti-inflammatory properties.
- Topically treats sunburn, minor burns, and helps with wound healing.
- Topically treats diabetic ulcers.
- Orally treats constipation but is a cause of melanosis coli (a brownish discoloration of the lining of the colon.

- Common dose: For constipation 50-200 mg per dose orally for a maximum of 10 days. For burns and sunburn aloe is very useful topically.
- Side effects: Rare but include allergic reactions to aloe. Commonly causes melanosis coli when taken internally.
- **My take: Excellent as a topical solution particularly for sunburn. If aloe vera is used for constipation it should only be taken for short periods of time.**
- **Rating: **** for skin use, *** for internal use**

Alpha-Lipoic Acid (Alpha-Linolenic Acid)

- Potent antioxidant and also potentiates the antioxidant effect of Vitamin C and E.
- Universal antioxidant as it is soluble in water and fat.
- Helps in glucose metabolism, liver detoxification, muscle energy, and neuropathies related to diabetes.
- Useful for improving visual function in glaucoma, improving glucose uptake in diabetics, and decreasing pain related to diabetic neuropathy.
- Some ALA is converted to EPA (a better form of Omega 3).
- Common dose: Glaucoma 150 mg per day, Diabetes 800 mg per day.
- Side effects: Rare but include skin rash and hypoglycemia (low blood sugar).
- **My take: EPA and DHA are more effective forms of Omega 3.**
- **Rating: *****

Quick tip

Building block antioxidants include the minerals Manganese, Zinc, Copper, Selenium .

Bee Pollen

- Natural antibiotic properties and stimulates the immune system.
- Helps with fatigue and decreases mucous membrane inflammation.
- **My take: May be useful for chronic fatigue.**
- **Rating: *****

Bilberry

- Excellent antioxidant properties with flavonoid.
- Improves retinal health in diabetics and may prevent cataracts and improve macular degeneration.
- Strengthens vascular walls and helps prevent atherosclerosis.
- Common dose: Extract 240 to 600 mg per day.
- Side effects: None reported.
- **My take: No major downside and may be useful in diabetics with eye disease.**
- **Rating: *****

Quick tip

Herbal antioxidants include Green Tea, Bilberry, Turmeric, and Ginkgo.

Blue Green Algae

- High in vitamins, minerals, protein, essential fatty acids, and carotenoids.
- Increases energy, improves the immune system, improves the thought process, decrease stress, and helps with insomnia.
- High doses may help with weight loss.
- Common dose: 2000 to 3000 mg per day in divided doses.
- Side effects: Minimal to none. Careful with heavy metals such as lead, mercury, or cadmium which may be in higher levels in the capsules as may contribute to heavy metal toxicity.
- **My take: No major risk and may be helpful in chronic fatigue.**
- **Rating: *****

Boswellia

- Active ingredient is terpenoids which have an anti-inflammatory effect.
- Helpful in Osteoarthritis and Rheumatoid arthritis. In some studies boswellia is as effective as nonsteroidal anti-inflammatory medications without the gastrointestinal side effects.
- Useful in cream form externally for muscle aches and bursitis.
- Common dose: 150 mg three times a day for up to 12 weeks. The cream can be purchased premade as used as needed.
- Side effects: Generally safe but occasionally diarrhea, skin rash, and nausea.
- **My take: Excellent choice for weekend athletes related muscle aches and pains. Use externally as a cream. Also very reasonable to try internally (in pill form) for inflammatory arthritis.**
- **Rating: ***** in cream form, *** in pill form**

Butterbur

- Anti-inflammatory properties on blood vessels.
- Helpful with migraines, hay fever, allergic rhinitis.

- Use only short term, preferably less than 2 weeks.
- **My take: No obviously down side. May be useful for environmental allergens.**
- **Rating: *****

Quick tip

Dangerous herbs include belladonna, bitter orange, chaparral, coltsfoot, comfrey, ephedra, germander, golden ragwort, goldenseal, kava, licorice root, lobelia, pennyroyal, Scotch broom, skullcap, wild ginger, and yohimbe. Avoid these herbal supplements.

Cat's Claw

- Treats inflammation even with Rheumatoid arthritis and Osteoarthritis and is the most common use.
- Improves the immune system and may be used in cancer patients and HIV.
- May decrease blood pressure.
- Common dose: 100 mg per day of a freeze-dried preparation.
- Side effects: Vaguely reported but should not be used in autoimmune illness, multiple sclerosis, tuberculosis, pregnancy, and if breast feeding.
- **My take: Consider this after Tumeric and Boswellia in the treatment of inflammatory arthritis.**
- **Rating: *****

Cayenne

- Found in red pepper and chili pepper.

- Active ingredient is capsaicin.
- Topically used for Rheumatoid arthritis and Osteoarthritis along with Diabetic Neuropathy.
- Orally useful for indigestion, gas and bloating, and Irritable Bowel Syndrome.
- May be useful in Diabetic Neuropathy.
- Common dose: Topically 0.025% to 75% capsaicin three to four times per day. Keep away from the eyes, mouth, and nose and do not put on open sores. Orally 833 mg capsule three times per day.
- Side effects: Minimal overall. Careful with the creams and eyes, etc. May increase GERD (acid reflux) and cause problems in patients with ulcer disease.
- **My take: No major downside, but beneficial treatment effects are not dramatic.**
- **Rating: *****

Chamomile

- Active ingredients include alpha-bisabolol oxides, matricin, flavonoids, and quercetin.
- Has anti-inflammatory, antispasmodic, and smooth muscle relaxing abilities, particularly in the gastrointestinal tract.
- Useful in Irritable Bowel Syndrome to control the gas, bloating, and abdominal cramps.
- Should only be used short term.
- Common dose: As a tea three to four times a day. 300 mg capsules three times a day. 3 to 4 ml of tincture three times a day.
- Side effects: Rare allergic reactions. Should not be used if allergic to ragweed, aster, or chrysanthemums.
- **My take: Very helpful for short term use in the gas and bloating associated with IBS.**
- **Rating: ******

Charcoal extract

- Antigas and antibacterial properties are helpful in Irritable Bowel Syndrome.

- Use on an as needed basis.
- Higher doses will cause black stools.
- May bind other medications and make them ineffective. Do not take charcoal extract within 2 hours of a prescription medication.
- Common dose: Standard tablets 1 to 2 as needed.
- Side effects: Minimal to none.
- **My take: Excellent for an as needed treatment for gas and bloating associated with IBS.**
- **Rating: ******

Chasteberry

- Useful in PMS symptoms including breast pain and tenderness, and mood changes.
- May be helpful in constipation.
- **My take: No obvious reason to avoid this supplement but certainly has unclear benefits. May try for premenstrual symptoms.**
- **Rating: *****

Cinnamon

- Use the water soluble extract. Terpenoids are the active ingredient.
- Improves sugar metabolism and is helpful in diabetic control particularly Type 2 Diabetes (Noninsulin).
- May help improve Irritable Bowel Syndrome and is useful in the treatment of diarrhea.
- Lowers cholesterol but requires higher doses.
- Common doses: Diabetics 1 gram per day, Cholesterol doses up to 6 grams per day.
- Side effects: Allergic reactions with bronchial constriction or skin rash. Use a small amount if never exposed to cinnamon in the past. If a known allergy exists then you should avoid this.
- **My take: Many potential benefits but most helpful for diarrhea associated with IBS.**

- Rating: ***

Quick tip

B Carotene is an antioxidant which in multiple studies has not shown great benefit in the prevention of cancer, heart disease, and inflammatory conditions.

Cod Liver Oil

- Anti-inflammatory properties and helps to fight infections.
- High in Omega 3, Vitamin A and Vitamin D. Do not take in combination with Vitamins A and D.
- Side effects: None.
- **My take: No down side outside of the lousy taste.**
- **Rating: ***

Devils Claw

- Active ingredients include harpagoside, harpagide, and procumbide.
- Anti-inflammatory agent which helps in Osteoarthritis and Low Back Pain.
- No evidence that it is helpful in Rheumatoid arthritis.
- Common dose: Standardized extract 1200 to 2500 mg per day.
- Side effects: Increases gastric acid secretion so do not use in patients with ulcer disease or GERD (reflux). Do not take if you have gallstones.
- **My take: May try after Tumeric, and Boswellia as an adjunctive treatment in inflammatory arthritis.**
- **Rating: ***

Dong Quai

- Unclear active ingredient.
- Generally used in combination with herbs such as peony and ligusticum.
- Referred to as the female ginsing as used in herbal combinations for abnormal menstrual cycles, abnormal menstrual bleeding, menstrual cramps, and menopausal symptoms.
- Common dose: 1 gram three times a day in capsules or tablets.
- Side effects: Sensitivity to sunlight in fair skinned people. Do not use in pregnancy or breast feeding.
- **My take: Reasonable to try in difficult to control menstrual symptoms.**
- **Rating: *****

Echinacea

- Antiviral and antibacterial properties which help in the common cold and flu.
- Stimulates the immune system.
- May increase the production of Interferon which has antiviral effects.
- Have been problems with quality control. Make sure you purchase a product with a quality seal.
- Unclear what is the active ingredient.
- May also be useful in bronchial, tonsillar, vaginal, and renal infections.
- Start at the onset of the symptoms. Does not appear to help in prevention of the common cold.
- Common dose: 300mg capsule or tablet every 2 hours for the first day then three times a day for 7-10 days.
- Side effects: Generally well tolerated but contraindicated in autoimmune disorders, lupus, tuberculosis, HIV, multiple sclerosis. Occasional cases of allergic reactions with diarrhea, wheezing, skin rash.
- **My take: Very popular for treatment of the common cold but I would prefer Andrographis.**
- **Rating: *****

Quick tip

Be careful with Echinacea intake in athletes who may be subject to drug tests. The medication may create a false positive test.

Elderberry Extract

- Antioxidant and antiviral effects.
- Treats the common cold and flu symptoms and may decrease the duration.
- Active ingredient is flavonoids with antioxidant effects and thereby anti-inflammatory effects.
- Common dose: 15 cc four times a day.
- Side effects: Safe use limited to dried flowers and ripe berry extract. The roots, stems, leaves, and unripe berries are poisonous and may cause nausea, vomiting, and diarrhea.
- **My take: Again, no major downside but I would prefer Andrographis.**
- **Rating: *****

Feverfew

- Active ingredient parthenolide which inhibits platelet aggregation and inhibits the release of serotonin and other inflammatory mediators.
- Relieves headache and migraine.
- Decreases fever.
- Anti-inflammatory effect on joints and treats arthritis.
- Best if used short term.

- Common dose: 6 mg per day.
- Side effects: Generally well tolerated but may cause gastrointestinal upset and nervousness.
- **My take: Useful for fever control.**
- **Rating: *****

Flaxseed and Flaxseed Oil

- Flaxseed is an excellent source of fiber, Omega 3 fatty acids (in the form of ALA or alpha linolenic acid), and lignans (produced in the gut by bacterial metabolism of flaxseed).
- Flaxseed oil contains Omega 3 but very little fiber and lignans.
- May have anti-inflammatory effects and decrease Triglyceride levels.
- Lignans have antioxidant activity and may help in the metabolism of estrogen.
- Common dose: Flaxseed- 1 tablespoon of whole or ground flaxseed twice a day. Take with a full glass of water. Flaxseed oil- 1 tablespoon per day. Flaxseed oil may be used in salads but is not suitable for cooking.
- Side effects: Minimal with occasional allergic reactions. Do not take if there is a possibility of bowel obstruction.
- **My take: Useful for the adjunctive treatment of elevated triglycerides.**
- **Rating: *****

Quick tip

Best antioxidant supplements include Omega-3, Coenzyme Q10, Flaxseed, Green tea, ALA and Pycnogenol.

Ginkgo Biloba

- Improves memory and mental fatigue.
- May be beneficial in macular degeneration and diabetic retinopathy.
- Antioxidant properties with flavonoids, terpenoids improve circulation and inhibit platelet aggregation.
- Do not use with blood thinners (anticoagulants) or aspirin.
- Do not take with thiazide diuretics and this may elevate blood pressure.
- Common dose: Standardized tablets with 120 to 240 mg per day. Higher doses used in Alzheimers and age related memory problems. May take 8-12 weeks to see a benefit.
- Side effects: May cause excessive bleeding so careful preoperatively. Tell your physicians if you are taking this medication. Occasional gastrointestinal upset and mild headaches.
- **My take: Reasonable supplement for the treatment of memory problems and to help maintain mental acuity. Be very careful with the bleeding problems associated with ginkgo.**
- **Rating: *****

Asian and American Ginsing

- Improves mental performance and decreases mental and physical fatigue.
- Increases testosterone levels and increase libido.
- Careful as may elevate the blood pressure.
- Use short term, up to 3 months.
- Common dose: 1-3 grams per day.
- Side effects: Insomnia and agitation.
- **My take: Reasonable supplement for memory problems and to help with mental acuity.**
- **Rating: *****

Gamma Linolenic Acid (GLA)

- Omega-6 fatty acid.

- Anti-inflammatory effects and may treat Rheumatoid arthritis, Ulcerative colitis, and Dermatitis.
- Best data is in the treatment of Diabetic neuropathy.
- Side effects: none.
- **My take: No specific downside but probably a waste of a supplement.**
- **Rating: *****

Quick tip

Excellent Irritable Bowel Syndrome options include Probiotics, Glutamine, Ginger, Peppermint, Melva tea, Slippery elm, and Chamomile.

Lecithan

- Emulsifies fat and therefore decreases cholesterol and triglycerides.
- May improve brain function.
- **My take: Probably another waste of a supplement, although not dangerous.**
- **Rating: *****

Melatonin

- Synthesized from tryptophan which by popular reports causes the sleepiness after eating turkey. In reality there is not enough tryptophan in turkey to put you to sleep. The lethargy after Thanksgiving dinner is related to the size of the meal.
- Improves sleep with chronic insomnia and jet lag.

- May be beneficial in stress, depression, migraines, and menopausal symptoms.
- Some studies suggest benefit in fibromyalgia.
- Use short term only.
- Many companies have produced Melatonin with essentially no melatonin in the product. Careful with what you purchase.
- Common dose: 1 to 3 mg per day
- Side effects: Minimal overall but drowsiness, sleepwalking, and disorientation have been reported. Vague reports of breast enlargement in men, loss of sex drive, and abdominal cramps.
- **My take: May be tried short term for insomnia related to stress.**
- **Rating: *****

Peppermint

- Contains a phytochemical called menthol which relaxes stomach muscle and improves bile flow.
- Helps with Irritable Bowel Syndrome, Dyspepsia, and Indigestion.
- Careful with GERD (Esophageal reflux) as may increase the symptoms.
- Should be used on an intermittant basis.
- Common dose: Enteric coated capsules- one capsule two to three times a day as needed.
- Side effects: Generally well tolerated. Careful with GERD and should not be taken if there are gallstones present. Do not use in infants.
- **My take: Very useful on an as needed treatment for the treatment of indigestion.**
- **Rating: ******

Senna

- Active ingredient is glycosides known as sennosides.

- Helpful with chronic constipation related to Irritable Bowel Syndrome or Colonic Inertia by stimulating colonic contractions.
- Common dose: Extract in capsules- 20-60 mg per day. May also take Senakot which is a brand name. Best is used short term- less than one week.
- Side effects: Colonic dependency on senna for contractions and subsequent bowel movement. A major cause of Melanosis coli which is a pigmentation change in the colon wall.
- **My take: Useful for acute, short term treatment of constipation. Do not use long term.**
- **Rating: *****

Quick tip

Senna is commonly the active ingredient in "herbal laxatives." Be careful with their long term use.

Slippery Elm Bark

- Active ingredient is the mucilage of the inner bark lining.
- Helpful in GERD (acid reflux) by providing a barrier against acid damage to the esophagus. Also has anti-inflammatory effects on the stomach and intestines which helps to treat diarrhea.
- May help with sore throats and is included in some throat lozenges.
- Common dose: 800 to 1000 mg in a capsule three to four times a day.
- Side effects: Generally well tolerated but may interfere with the absorption of medications. Should be used short term.
- **My take: If other treatment options fail, may use this supplement in the treatment of diarrhea and GERD.**
- **Rating: *****

St Johns Wort

- Active ingredient is hypericin, flavonoids, xanthones, and hyperforin.
- Treats mild to moderate depression and anxiety.
- Used topically to treat burns and wounds.
- Common dose: 500 to 1000 mg per day as a capsule of extract.
- Side effects: Generally well tolerated with occasional gastrointestinal upset, fatigue, sleep disturbance, skin rash, and itching. Careful with interactions with antidepressants, birth control pills, anticoagulation medications, steroids, and asthma medications.
- **My take: Helpful for the treatment of depression. St. Johns Wort may interact with anesthesia medications so if you are undergoing surgery be sure to stop this supplement 1 week in advance and make sure you inform your physicians, including the anesthesiologist.**
- **Rating: ******

Quick tip

St. Johns Wort may precipitate a manic episode in patients with bipolar disorder and should be avoided in this group.

Valarian Root

- Unclear active ingredient but may be volatile oils.

- Helpful for sleep disorder, insomnia, anxiety.
- Treats abdominal cramping associated with Irritable Bowel Syndrome.
- Common dose: 300 to 500 mg in concentrated extract capsules. Use before bedtime or as needed for abdominal cramps.
- Side effects: Minimal overall. Does not appear to impair driving ability.
- **My take: May consider for short term treatment of insomnia.**
- **Rating: *****

White Willow Bark

- Anti-inflammatory effects and treats low back pain.
- Common dose: 400 mg per day.
- **My take: Many other excellent supplements should be tried first.**
- **Rating: *****

Quick tip

Tell your physician about all herbal and natural supplements you are taking. This is particularly important before surgery as many supplements interact with anesthesia and may cause increased bleeding during surgery.

Popular but questionable Supplements

Hawthorne

- Antioxidant with flavenoids.
- Dilates blood vessels and improves overall blood flow. May treat Congestive Heart Failure and improve Angina.
- Lowers blood pressure to a small degree.
- Common dose: Herbal extract in capsules with 80-300 mg two to three times per day. Slow acting and takes time to work.
- Side effects: Data is scarce and unclear as to the potential for severe side effects.
- **My take: Avoid this supplement.**
- **Rating: ****

Hoodia

- Used as an appetite suppressant by stimulating the hypothalamus as making your body believe it is full.
- Not much data available and unclear if it is safe.
- **My take: Currently very popular but with many questions. I would avoid.**
- **Rating: ****

Licorice

- Active ingredient are flavonoids and glycyrrhizin.
- Used primarily for ulcer disease and may kill the ulcer forming bacteria called H. pylori.
- Has also been used for Chronic fatigue syndrome and Respiratory infections.
- Common dose: Concentrated extract 250 to 500 mg two to three times a day for chronic fatigue. De-glycyrrhizinated (DGL) used for ulcer disease with 200 to 300 mg four times a day.
- Side effects: Significant problems with blood pressure elevation and water retention primarily related to compounds containing glycyrrhizin. DGL

compounds may increase GERD (reflux) and counteract other medical treatment. Overall would use with extreme caution and only short term.
- **My take: Way too many potential medical side effects.**
- **Rating: ***

Noni Juice

- Active ingredient probably polysaccharides and damnacanthal.
- Plenty of advertisement with multiple claims including use in arthritis, diabetes, high blood pressure, pain control, diarrhea, cancer, AIDS, etc.
- No convincing data on anything.
- Common dose: 4 oz before breakfast or in extract capsules 500 to 1000 mg per day
- Side effects: Does not appear dangerous in lower doses.
- **My take: Another popular supplement with questionable benefits. Don't waste your money.**
- **Rating: ****

DHEA

- Billed as an anti-aging supplement that increases muscle, decreases body fat, elevates sex drive, and increases memory.
- Multiple articles and books written in support.
- Many serious side effects with higher doses.
- Has been banned from competitive sports.
- **My take: Acceptable to use in low doses (25-50mg per day). I have personally diagnosed way too many problems when high doses are used.**
- **Rating: *** in low doses * in high doses**

Dangerous Supplements

Ephedra (Ma Huang)

- Includes Ephedrine and Pseudoephedrine.
- Used for weight loss particularly in combination with caffeine.
- Useful for colds, bronchitis, asthma.
- Unclear if there are multiple heart related deaths from ephedra but the cardiac risk does appear to be significant. Easily will raise the blood pressure with multiple potential problems. Would avoid this if possible.
- **My take: Avoid.**
- **Rating: ***

Goldenseal

- Multiple claims including stimulating the immune system, treating colds and flu, helping digestive problems, and treating infectious diarrhea.
- Active ingredient is berberine.
- At best should be used short term (less than one week) but has had serious side effects reported.
- Do not use with ragweed allergy.
- Common dose: Standardized extracts 250 to 500 mg three times a day.
- Side effects: Serious gastrointestinal and nervous system effects may occur. This is a particular problem with higher doses and for longer periods of time.
- **My take: Not worth the risk particularly with the minimal beneficial effects.**
- **Rating: ***

Quick tip

Goldenseal does not hide the detection of illicit drugs in drug tests as is popular to report.

Kava

- Used for stress and anxiety as it acts as a sedative and muscle relaxant
- Many cases of liver failure reported
- Should not be used. Has been banned in many countries
- **My take: Avoid at all costs.**
- **Rating: ***

Mistletoe

- Used in Europe as an anticancer drug but incorrect use can be poisonous.
- American mistletoe is more toxic than European mistletoe.
- Induce vomiting if accidental ingestion occurs particularly with children at Christmas time.
- **My take: Avoid.**
- **Rating: ***

CAM (Complementary and Alternative Medicine) and Common Diseases

Complementary and alternative medicine can be valuable in a variety of medical conditions although commonly these treatment protocols have not been proven scientifically (through double blind studies and statistical analysis) to be beneficial. Integrative Medicine takes this into consideration and evaluates which CAM treatment regiments clinically make sense and are scientifically intellectually reasonable. This thought process is not designed to believe all claims made by the manufacturers of these supplements, but to realize that many complementary treatments are useful. Integrative medicine helps sort out the ridiculous statements will be advertised in the interest of selling the product.

Alzheimer's Disease

- **Dietary changes**: Consider decreasing aluminum intake by reducing contact with aluminum (aluminum pots, aluminum foil, aluminum cans), avoiding aluminum containing foods (American cheese, chocolate pudding, chocolate beverages, salt, and some chewing gum), avoiding medications with aluminum (Amphogel, Alternagel), and careful with aluminum added to municipal water (bottled water in these areas).
- **Keep active physically and mentally**: Art or music therapy has been shown to be very beneficial.
- **Nutritional treatment**: Salmon or Spanish mackerel for the high Omega-3 levels. Salmon is also high in niacin which may help in Alzheimer's. Blueberries have high antioxidants which may help decrease the risk of Alzheimer's.
- **Acetyl-L-Carnitine**: 1 gram three times a day may be beneficial.
- **Vitamin B1, Vitamin B6, Vitamin C, and Vitamin E:** Supplementation may be beneficial therefore a Super B Vitamin daily is an excellent choice.
- **Coenzyme Q10:** 100 mg per day.
- **Omega-3**: EPA and DHA supplementation with at least 600 mg per day.

- **Ginkgo Biloba:** 120 mg to 240 mg per day is the standard dose but higher doses are commonly needed for Alzheimer's disease. Remember it commonly takes 8-12 weeks to see any benefit.
- **Choline:** 400 mg choline alfoscerate three times a day. This supplement may improve your bodies ability to transmit nerve signals in the brain.
- ➤ **My take:** Dietary changes (decreasing aluminum intake), keeping active physically and mentally (extremely important), and Omega 3 supplementation all make sense with a minimal down side. Taking a multiple vitamin and a super B complex vitamin is recommended for everyone on a regular basis, including Alzheimer's patients. Ginkgo biloba may help middle aged people with concentration problems, but is less likely to make a major difference in a person with Alzheimer's disease.

Quick tip

Before embarking on CAM therapy, make sure that the patient has been carefully evaluated from a neurological standpoint to rule out treatable causes of dementia.

Arthritis

- **Tumeric:** 250 mg to 500 mg three times a day. The anti-inflammatory effects are similar to COX 2 inhibitors (Celebrex).
- **Glucosamine with/without Chondroitin and MSM:** 1000 mg – 2000 mg per day (of the Glucosamine component) in divided doses. This supplement is considered very helpful for mild to moderate degenerative joint disease/osteoarthritis but is not beneficial in severe inflammatory diseases such as rheumatoid arthritis.
- **SAMe:** 800 mg- 1200 mg per day. Useful in mild joint inflammation.
- **Boswellia:** Orally for osteoarthritis and rheumatoid arthritis. Topically for muscle and joint aches and pains.
- **Cats Claw:** 100 mg per day. It may be effective in osteoarthritis and rheumatoid arthritis.

- **Cayenne**: Topically used for osteoarthritis and rheumatoid arthritis.
- **Devils Claw**: 1200 mg- 2500 mg per day. Used in the treatment of osteoarthritis and low back pain.
- **White Willow Bark**: 400 mg per day. Considered helpful for low back pain.
- **Acupuncture:** This form of treatment must be done on a regular schedule to be valuable long term. It can end up being expensive but is very effective.

➢ **My take:** Tumeric is worth a try in arthritis particularly if there is an inflammatory component. Glucosamine with Chondroitin and MSM is very useful in the regular mild to moderate joint aches and pains we all experience with aging, but is not helpful in true inflammatory arthritis (particularly rheumatoid arthritis). Boswellia is most useful for short term topical use for acute muscle aches and pains particularly for the weekend athlete. Acupuncture is very useful but requires several treatments and is more expensive.

Atherosclerosis (Coronary artery disease)/Heart disease

- **Dietary changes** with low fat and low sodium diet (a no added salt is approximately 4 grams of NaCl (salt) per day):
- **Diets high in the antioxidant Alpha-linolenic acid** are beneficial: ALA found in Canola oil and Flaxseed. Also diets with beans, peas, fish, vegetables, and fruit are helpful in controlling and preventing heart disease.
- **Dietary fiber** with higher amounts of whole wheat products, oats, and psyllium.
- **Weight loss:** Clearly needs to be maintained on a long term basis.
- **Exercise:** This needs to be done on a regular schedule for optimum results.
- **Omega-3**: Excellent data supporting the chronic use. 1500 mg per day total dose with 600 mg per day of DHA and EPA.
- **Coenzyme Q10**: 100 mg per day assists with decreasing platelet aggregation.
- **Arginine**: 3 grams to 5 grams per day. This is an amino acid which causes nitrous oxide formation which allow for dilation of the heart blood vessels. This permits a more effective exercise regiment.

- **Green tea:** One cup daily.
- **Cod liver oil**
- ➤ **My take:** Clearly dietary changes with low fat, low salt, high fiber, fruits, vegetables, and whole wheat products are very important. Weight loss and exercise are equally important to dietary treatment. Adding extra Omega 3 with supplements or diet (cold water fish) is clearly beneficial. Coenzyme Q10 and Green tea may also be helpful.

Quick tip

Vitamin E has not shown any significant benefit in heart disease and already has fallen out of favor.

Attention Deficit- Hyperactivity Disorder (ADHD)

- **Feingold diet**: This diet eliminates additives and foods including dyes such as yellow dye tartazine which may cause problems.
- **L- Carnitine**: 100 mg per kilogram (2.2 pounds per kg) with a maximum of 4 grams per day.
- **Magnesium supplements**: 200 mg per day which is particularly helpful if magnesium deficiency exists.
- **Fatty Acid supplementation: Omega-3** with EPA and DHA (600 mg per day). Also consider adding GLA (gamma- linolenic acid).
- **Zinc**: 15 mg per day may be beneficial.
- **Vitamin B6** supplementation: Requires higher doses 15-30 mg/kg/day.
- **Ginkgo and Ginseng combination:** 50 mg of ginkgo and 200 mg of Asian or American ginseng in a combination and take twice a day.
- Another reason to **avoid smoking** during pregnancy as this may increase the risk of ADHD in the unborn child.
- ➤ **My take:** This is a difficult problem to treat but the Feingold diet and Zinc supplementation are helpful. Omega 3 supplements and a Super B

vitamin should be taking daily in normal circumstances and are even more important with ADHD.

Chronic Fatigue Syndrome

- **Dietary changes**: Be extra careful with refined sugars.
- **Nutritional treatment**: Green tea contains antioxidants which increase metabolism. Diets higher in protein also increase the energy level.
- **Exercise frequently**: Best choice would be aerobic exercise sessions 4-6 times per week with anaerobic sessions 3-4 times per week.
- **Massage**: This form of treatment much be done regularly and would be fairly expensive. My suggestion would be weekly to a minimum of biweekly.
- **Vitamin B12**: Injections monthly of 1000 mcg of B12 can provide an energy boost particularly for the several days after the injection. B12 is a water soluble vitamin therefore any excess will be excreted through the kidneys.
- **Super B complex vitamin**: One per day.
- **Magnesium supplements**: 200 mg per day is particularly beneficial if the magnesium level is low.
- **Omega-3**: Particularly combinations of EPA and DHA, 600 mg per day.
- **L-Carnitine**: 1gram three times a day has been beneficial in one study.
- **Ginseng**: 100 mg to 200 mg of panex ginseng daily.
- Consider: **Art therapy, music therapy, meditation, and yoga.**
- ➤ **My take:** Avoid refined sugars as this is an extremely important dietary adjustment. Continue with a regular weekly exercise regiment. Use meditation to help control stress as this exacerbates chronic fatigue. Finally daily Omega 3 and Super B complex supplementation is recommended with a consideration of monthly B12 injections by your physician. Magnesium supplements if your magnesium level is low.

Quick tip

Licorice and DHEA have been reported to be beneficial in chronic fatigue but have potentially serious side effects.

Common Cold

- **Andrographis**: 100 mg twice a day in a standard extract or 500 mg- 3000 mg three times a day if the dried herb is used. If taken early it appears to decrease the duration and severity of symptoms. An excellent prep is Kan Jang which also contains ginsing.
- **Echinacea**: 300 mg every 2 hours the first day, then 300 mg three times a day for 7-10 days. Do not use Echinacea long term. Overall mixed data on the efficacy, but may decrease the duration and severity of symptoms.
- **Garlic**: 600 mg- 900 mg of the enteric coated capsules 2-3 times a day. There is minimal data to suggest it is beneficial in viruses, but chronic use may decrease the frequency of colds.
- **Vitamin C**: 500 mg- 2000 mg per day. It is most useful in extreme athletes such as marathon and ultramarathon runners. For most people, the benefit is not clear despite the extensive press. Despite this, Vitamin C is very safe as is it water soluble and any excess not needed by your body will be excreted by the kidney preventing any potential harmful effects.
- **Zinc lozenges**: 25mg per day. This helps stop the progression of symptoms and shorten the illness.
- **Feverfew**: 6 mg per day. Helpful with both headaches and fevers.
- **Elderberry extract:** 15 cc (milliliters) four times a day.
- **Bee Pollen**: This is particularly useful for mucous membrane inflammation.

- **Nutritional treatment**: Green tea contains a chemical, EGCG, that prevents the adenovirus from replicating. Oranges contain high levels of zinc and Vitamin C.
- ➤ **My take**: Rest, plenty of fluid intake, and chicken soup form the basis for treatment of the common cold. Andrographis and Zinc will decrease the severity of symptoms and shorten the duration. Although very popular Echinacea does not appear to have a beneficial effect on the common cold. For competitive athletes remember that Echinacea may create a false positive drug screen. Extreme athletes should consider high dose Vitamin C.

Quick tip

Don't forget the basics in treatment of the common cold including rest, plenty of fluids, and chicken soup. Believe it or not, scientific benefit has been shown with chicken soup!!!

Constipation

- **Fluids and Exercise**: Overall this is very important and forms the foundation of constipation treatment.
- **Dietary changes with high fiber**: Whole wheat products, fruits, and vegetables all on a daily basis.
- **Probiotics**: 2-30 billion bacteria per day. (around 10 billion is an excellent goal) This is helpful with both constipation and diarrhea. The probiotics should be taken daily, long term basis for the maximum benefit.

- **Fiber supplements**: The dose depends on what fiber supplement is used but generally once or twice a day is an excellent choice. When hard stools are a problem, fiber helps hold water in the colon and softens the bowel movement. My personal favorite is Benefiber as this dissolves very well in any fluid, can be placed on cereal or other foods, and even can be mixed in the prune juice. It is essentially tasteless!!
- **Prune Juice**: 4 oz once or twice a day. This is particularly effective when combined with fiber. Be careful if you are a diabetic as this does contain moderate amounts of sugar.
- **Garlic**: 600 mg- 900 mg 2-3 times a day of the enteric coated tablets.
- **Rhubarb**
- **Aloe Vera**: 50 mg- 200 mg per dose as needed. Do not use continuously for more than 10 days. It is important to be very careful with colonic dependence as aloe vera causes colonic stimulation which will result in your colon requiring higher doses over time to obtain the same result. Melanosis coli will eventually develop which is a brownish discoloration in the lining of the colon.
- **Senna**: Senakot 2 tablets as needed for acute constipation. Again, you must be cautious with chronic use as it causes colonic stimulation and colonic dependence. Therefore would only use senna for short periods of time. This also is a cause of Melanosis Coli. Be careful with the category of "Herbal laxatives" as commonly the active ingredient is senna.
- **Flaxseed**: 1 tsp to 2 tsp of freshly ground seeds and sprinkle on cereal or a salad.
- **Milk of Magnesia**: 2 tbsp twice a day as needed. This is an excellent prep to use for constipation. Generally I suggest using this as needed but occasionally is helpful in low doses on a daily basis.
- ➢ **My take**: Simple treatment generally works very well if it is used on a daily basis. Start with plenty of fluid intake and a weekly exercise program. Exercise promotes colonic motility and assists with the excretion of magnesium in the bowel movements both of which help to promote normal stools. A high fiber diet and daily probiotics are also very beneficial. Fiber supplements (many excellent available but my preference is Benefiber) with or without daily prune juice (4 oz once or twice a day) are helpful.

Quick tip

Swiss Criss is a favorite over the counter laxative which contains senna and will cause melanosis coli. Try to avoid laxatives that are stimulants to the colon (like senna) as they will require higher doses over time to achieve the same response.

Diabetes

- **Multivitamin daily along with nutritional support**: Overall will help decrease the risk of infection.
- **Dietary changes**: Carefully adhering to a diabetic diet is crucial to wellness. Eat 4-6 small "meals" per day with low fat and high fiber.
- **Fiber supplementation**: May help control glucose level. My personal favorite is Benefiber once or twice a day.
- **Weight loss and exercise**: As always, these are extremely important.
- **Chromium picolinate**: 200 mcg- 400 mcg per day. Supplement which may improve glucose sensitivity and thereby improve diabetic control.
- **Alpha-lipoic acid**: Appears to improve insulin sensitivity which permits easier glucose control.
- **Cinnamon**: Another supplement designed to improve glucose control.
- **Coenzyme Q 10**: 100 mg per day. This supplement is an antioxidant which helps control glucose levels and decreases the risks of high blood pressure.
- **Cayenne (capsaisin) ointment**: May apply this topically for the discomfort associated with diabetic neuropathy.
- **Multiple supplements and herbs** described including Fenugreek, Magnesium, Zinc, L-Carnitine, Vitamins B and C, Ginsing, and Bilberry all of which have been reported to improve diabetic control.
- ➢ **My take:** Certainly weight loss and weight control, nutrition with a proper diabetic diet, a multiple vitamin with minerals daily, and exercise form the

foundation of the treatment of diabetes. Chromium picolinate would be a reasonable addition for the potential added benefit of glucose control. CAM therapy does not substitute for appropriate diabetic control by your physician.

Diarrhea

- **Probiotic**: 2-30 billion bacteria per day (10 billion is an excellent goal) is an extremely useful adjunctive treatment for diarrhea. This will be beneficial for multiple etiologies of the diarrhea and helps dramatically for the gas and bloating associated with gastrointestinal problems.
- **Dietary changes with high fiber:** Increase the fiber in your diet with whole wheat products, fruits, and vegetables. These are healthy from an overall wellness standpoint and are very healthy for your intestines.
- **Glutamine**: 5 grams- 15 grams twice a day. This is an amino acid which repairs intestinal tissue and also helpful with the treatment of infectious diarrhea.
- **Fiber supplements**: All fiber will help absorb excess water in the colon and thereby decrease the frequency and intensity of the diarrhea. My personal favorite in chronic diarrhea is Fibercon (or the generic equivalent) which in normal situations has a tendency to cause constipation. A close second choice is Benefiber.
- **Zinc**: 15 mg- 25 mg daily. Clearly helps to repair intestinal tissue, both in the colon and small bowel.
- **Ginger/Valarian/Chamomile**: Supplements that are helpful with abdominal cramps associated with the intestinal contractions from the diarrhea.
- **Cinnamon**: May be used for the treatment of acute or chronic diarrhea.
- **Charcoal**: 2 pills 2-3 times per day. Be careful to use this short term (less than 3 days) as it can interfere with intestinal absorption. The charcoal will turn your stools black. There is some thought that this has some degree of anti-bacterial activity in addition to binding toxins in the colon.
- **Melva tea**: Useful for short periods of time for diarrhea and abdominal cramping.
- **Slippery Elm Bark**: This herb has an anti-inflammatory effect on the intestines and is helpful in treating diarrhea.

- **Cayenne capsules**: Oral tablets or the powdered form may help with digestion by assisting in the breakdown of food constituents.
- **Consider superimposed Lactose Intolerance** in patients with chronic diarrhea. This responds well to a lactose free diet or lactaid tablets taken before the intake of milk sugar (lactose).
- ➤ **My take:** Chronic diarrhea treatment should start with dietary changes as many different foods or the additives in foods may precipitate diarrhea. The foods will vary from patient to patient and may require a food diary to help determine the problem. Lactose (milk sugar) intolerance is common and should always be considered as it is simple to treat. The second line of treatment includes a high fiber diet, adding a fiber supplement, and taking a probiotic on a daily basis. Infectious diarrhea and Inflammatory bowel disease treatment is assisted with glutamine and zinc. Irritable bowel syndrome cramps and bloating are treated with ginger and chamomile.

Quick tip

Chronic changes in bowel habits require medical evaluation, particularly if there is a recent change. Other "red flag" symptoms include GI bleeding, weight loss, and nocturnal (nighttime) symptoms.

Dyslipidemia: Hypercholesterolemia and/or Hypertriglyceridemia

- **Low fat diet and Exercise:** These are crucial in dyslipidemia treatment.
- **Fiber:** Particularly whole wheat or oatmeal are slightly beneficial.
- **Omega-3**: 1500 mg per day with at least 600 mg of EPA and DHA although some patients require up to 4 grams per day. Fish oil is particularly beneficial in the treatment of a high triglyceride level with and

additional benefit of elevating the HDL (good cholesterol). Omega 3 supplementation will lower cholesterol/LDL to some degree.

- **Red Yeast Rice**: Works as a pre statin drug and helps lower cholesterol and to a lesser degree triglycerides. Like statins, red yeast rice has a small potential for causing liver disease and serum liver tests should be monitored intermittently (every 3-6 months).
- **Garlic**: Regular garlic tablet intake will improve cholesterol and to a small degree, triglycerides.
- **Flaxseed**: Chronic intake of flaxseed with help decrease the triglyceride levels.
- **Lecithan**: This supplement will lower cholesterol and triglycerides to some degree.
- ➤ **My take**: Dietary changes with a low fat diet and exercise are the foundation of treating dyslipidemias. Omega 3 is particularly helpful for a high triglyceride level but should be taken by all patients. Red yeast rice is beneficial in high cholesterol levels.

Fibromyalgia

- **Acupuncture**: Potentially acupuncture is very beneficial but needs to be done on a regular schedule. Single acupuncture treatments are not efficacious. This treatment can be expensive.
- **Massage**: Also requires multiple session for maximum benefit although occasionally single treatments will be helpful. Massage will help relax muscles and treat chronic pain. With multiple sessions can be expensive.
- **SAMe**: 800 mg twice a day. This supplement can be beneficial with its broad anti-inflammatory effect and is valuable in the treatment of myalgias and arthralgias associated with fibromyalgia.
- **5-HTP** (hydroxytryptophane): 100mg three times a day.
- **Coenzyme Q 10:** 100 mg per day. Antioxidant effect helps protect cells and may help improve oxygen supplies to cells.
- **American or Asian Ginseng:** 100 mg twice a day. This is beneficial for sleep and stress management in addition to increasing energy levels.
- **Stress management, good sleep habits, and regular exercise.**
- ➤ **My take:** The foundation of the treatment of fibromyalgia involves stress management with regular sleep habits and regular exercise.

Acupuncture and massage are great if you can afford them. SAMe is a cost effective treatment which commonly is beneficial.

Headache

- **Acupuncture:** This treatment is very efficacious in chronic headache conditions.
- **Biofeedback:** Beneficial as it teaches how to monitor and control certain physical responses.
- **Massage:** Helpful in the treatment of chronic headaches.
- **Stress management, good sleep habits, and regular exercise.**
- **Hypnosis:** Treatment technique which is also very beneficial for chronic headaches.
- **Feverfew:** Cost effective supplement which treats headaches and fevers.
- **Butterbur**
- **Willow bark:** 240 mg per day. Useful as a pain relieving medication but may be associated with rebound headaches after discontinuance.
- **Vitamins: Riboflavin (B2):** Easy treatment option as a super B vitamin supplement should be used on a daily basis for all patients.
- **Magnesium supplements:** This supplement is particularly helpful if there is and underlying magnesium deficiency.
- **Nutritional treatment:** Healthy fats in olive oil and avocados help decrease inflammation which may promote migraines.
- ➤ **My take:** Start with a super B complex like you should be taking on a daily basis. Feverfew is a cost effective second choice particularly if it is only needed for a relatively short time. If you can afford massage and/or acupuncture they are quite helpful. Massage is best in chronic muscle tension problems and acupuncture is helpful in most situations. Don't forget the foundation with stress management, regular sleep habits, and exercise.

Quick tip

Chronic headaches, particularly with early AM symptoms and blurred vision, may indicate significant CNS (brain) problems and require a physician's evaluation. New onset severe headaches should always be evaluated by a physician.

Indigestion/GERD (Heartburn)

- **Eat slowly** with smaller more frequent meals (5-6 small "meals" per day).
- **Watch for lactose intolerance and other dietary problems.** You may need to use a diet diary to determine foods that are precipitating symptoms.
- **Lactase tablets**: 2-3 tablets before meals. These simple supplements are quite beneficial in lactose intolerance. The tablets are taken before lactose ingestion and provide the lactase necessary for digestion.
- **Pancreatic enzyme supplements**: 2-3 tablets before meals to aid in digestion.
- Herbal treatment includes Bitters (digestive stimulants), Carminatives (gas-relieving), and Demulcents (soothing herbs)
- **Bitters: Andrographis, dandelion, and devil's claw.**
- **Carminatives: Chamomile, cinnamon, fennel, ginger, peppermint, and turmeric.**
- **Demulcents: Marshmellow (melva tea), and slippery elm.**
- ➢ **My take:** This is an area with multiple options as the symptoms can be extremely variable. The foundation involves eating smaller, more frequent meals and take your time eating. If lactose intolerance is a problem this should be treated with a lactose free diet and/or lactaid tablets. Peppermint is very valuable when gas, bloating, and indigested are the prominent symptoms but may increase heartburn problems so be careful if there is superimposed GERD. Chamomile is very helpful with gas and bloating. Slippery elm is useful in chronic indigestion.

Insomnia

- Insure a **quiet room** with a comfortable mattress to promote a good night's sleep.
- **Careful with stimulants** such as caffeine, ephedra, and pseudoephredrine. Try to eliminate or as a minimum decrease the intake.
- **Relaxation**: To assist with relaxation, consider meditation during times of stress.
- **Valarian**: 300 to 600mg before bedtime.
- **Melatonin:** Nightly use a melatonin for sleep is one of the original herbal supplements that hit the market.
- **5-HTP** (hydroxytryptophan).
- **Nutritional treatment:** Nonfat popcorn will help your body create serotonin, a chemical which causes relaxation. Sesame seeds are high in tryptophan which helps induce sleep. Bananas and walnuts are high in melatonin which is a hormone that induces sleep.
- ➤ **My take:** Start with a quiet room, no stimulants, and relaxation. Generally avoiding TV after going to bed is considered best, but many people will fall asleep easier if they are watching TV. Each person needs to determine what works best for them. Even a warm glass of milk at bedtime may be valuable. If this is not sufficient try melatonin.

Irritable Bowel Syndrome/Gas/Bloating

- **Probiotics**: Very beneficial for the treatment of gas, bloating, abdominal cramps, diarrhea, and constipation when taken on a regular basis.
- **Glutamine**: Can repair intestinal tissue and treats diarrhea. This is most useful for infectious diarrhea.
- **Fiber supplements**: Daily fiber supplementation is very helpful in the treatment of IBS. My personal favorite is Benefiber as it is very useful for multiple IBS symptoms.
- **Peppermint**: Very helpful on an as needed basis for abdominal cramps, gas, and bloating but be careful as peppermint can increase heartburn (GERD).
- **Chamomile**: This supplement should only be used short term for gas, bloating, and abdominal cramps.
- **Charcoal**: 2-3 tablets 2-3 times a day for a maximum of 3 consecutive days. Another supplement which should only be used short term as needed for gas and bloating.

- **Valerian root, Melva tea, and Ginger**: All three herbal supplements are used for abdominal cramps.
- **Cinnamon**: Most commonly suggested for the treatment of diarrhea.
- **Slippery elm**: Has an anti-inflammatory effect on the intestines.
- **Digestive enzymes**: 1-2 tablets before each meal. Most beneficial for gas, bloating, and diarrhea.
- **Acupuncture**: This treatment can be extremely beneficial in the treatment of IBS. Acupuncture must be used on a regular basis for the maximum benefit.
- **Biofeedback, exercise, massage, meditation, yoga, stress management, and hypnosis** are all beneficial.
- ➤ **My take:** IBS has many different symptoms including diarrhea, constipation, alternating diarrhea and constipation, abdominal pain, bloating, etc. The treatment options vary based on the symptoms. The foundation of treatment includes stress management (meditation and/or yoga are excellent choices), exercise, dietary manipulation, fiber, and probiotics. Peppermint and Chamomile are helpful on an as needed basis for gas, bloating, and indigestion but be careful if heartburn (GERD) is a problem. Slippery elm should be tried in recurrent, difficult situations. Acupuncture is an excellent option if the higher cost is acceptable.

Menopausal Symptoms

- **Soy**: Commonly this treatment is very effective for hot flashes, headaches, and mood disorders associated with menopause.
- **Black Cohash**: This herbal supplement is also used for hot flashes, headaches, and mood disorders. It should not be used continuously for more than 3-6 months.
- **Dong Quai**: May be helpful for both menopausal and menstrual symptoms.
- **Ginsing**: This treats mood and sleep disorders but is not effective for hot flashes.
- **Acupuncture**: Regular treatment sessions are very effective.
- **Yoga, stress management, meditation, regular sleep patterns, and deep breathing** are all beneficial.
- ➤ **My take:** The foundation is formed with stress management (meditation and/or yoga are excellent choices), and a regular sleep pattern. Soy is a

very good first treatment choice and black cohash may be added for 3-6 months. Acupuncture is an excellent choice is the cost is acceptable.

Nausea and Vomiting

- **Acupuncture and Acupressure**
- **Ginger:** This supplement is particularly helpful with motion sickness, pregnancy, post anesthesia, and chemotherapy.
- ➤ **My take:** This is a difficult problem to treat. Ginger should be tried first but acupuncture is generally very beneficial. Acupuncture must be used on a regular basis.

PMS: Premenstrual Syndrome

- **Magnesium:** 400mg per day. Magnesium supplements can help with fluid retention, breast tenderness, and bloating.
- **Vitamin B6:** 50 to 100mg per day. Supplement that is effective for varied PMS symptoms.
- **Black Cohash:** Helps to control menstrual cramps, but again use less than 3-6 months on a continuous basis.
- **Chasteberry:** This supplement is useful for breast tenderness, mood changes, and headaches.
- **Dong Quai:** May be used intermittently for menstrual cramps
- **Ginkgo:** Regular use helps to control breast tenderness.
- **Acupuncture**
- ➤ **My take:** Make sure you a taking a Super B complex as this will start your B6 supplementation. Magnesium supplementation during your menstrual cycle is beneficial. Black cohash may be used for short periods during times of significant PMS flares.

Prostate Health

- **Exercise and weight loss** is very beneficial. Overweight men have an increased risk of prostate cancer.
- **Saw Palmetto:** This is a classical herbal treatment that is very helpful.

- **Beta-sitosterol and Rye pollen**: May be used to improve urine flow.
- Prevention of Prostate Cancer with **Selenium** (200mcg per day), **Lycopene** (found in tomatoes or capsule form 15mg twice a day), **Vitamins D and E.**
- ➤ **My take:** Exercise, weight loss, and regular lycopene form the foundation of preventative prostate treatment. Saw palmetto should be tried when symptoms of BPH (Benign Prostatic Hypertrophy) occur. BPH symptoms are most commonly a decrease in the urine flow or incomplete emptying of the bladder.

Quick tip

Be sure there is adequate evaluation for prostate cancer as this can mimic BPH. A blood test measuring the PSA level is an excellent screening technique.

Sexual Problems

- **Acupuncture**
- **Ginkgo**: 120 mg to 240 mg twice a day. This herb increases penile blood flow and improves depression.
- **Asian Ginseng**: 100 mg to 200 mg per day. Can be useful for decreased libido and for erectile dysfunction.
- **L-Arginine**: 3 grams to 5 grams per dose and may also be used daily. Nitrous oxide stimulant which improves penile blood flow.
- **DHEA**: Lower doses (25-50mg per day) are reasonable but use caution with higher doses as there are many potential significant problems.
- ➤ **My take**: Very difficult problem but daily DHEA in low doses is reasonable.

Quick tip

Use extreme caution with DHEA, Yohimba Bark Extract, and Herbal Viagra's as there are many potential serious side effects. Yohimba in particular helps with erectile dysfunction but with potential problems.

Stress, Anxiety, and Depression

- **St Johns Wort**: This herbal supplement is very beneficial for stress and anxiety, and is also helpful with depression which commonly coexists.
- **Valerian**: Also useful for sleep disorders including insomnia.
- **Super B complex vitamin:** One per day.
- **Omega 3:** 1500 mg per day with 600 mg of this EPA and DHA. This supplement is particularly useful for depression.
- **SAMe:** 800 mg twice a day. Has been helpful particularly in depression.
- **Massage**
- **Relaxation techniques**
- **Yoga**
- **Biofeedback**
- **Consider: Acupuncture, aromatherapy, art therapy, and music therapy**
- **Nutritional treatment:** 1 tbsp of ground flaxseed contains ALA (alpha-linoleic acid) which helps the cerebral cortex induce pleasure feelings. High Omega-3 fish such as salmon, Spanish mackerel, and Halibut help with depression. Arugula and spinach are excellent sources of B vitamins which treat depression. Red bell peppers are high in Vitamin C which helps decrease the release of stress hormones. Sesame seeds are high in magnesium which assists with stress coping abilities. Peppermint tea helps you focus during times of stress. Situational anxiety may be treated with lysine (yogurt is high in lysine) or arginine (nuts are high in arginine).

> ➢ **My take:** Relaxation techniques with meditation and yoga in particular form the foundation of stress and anxiety treatment. Make sure you take your Super B complex vitamin. Although difficult, try to control the underlying problems creating the stress. St. Johns Wort is an excellent choice for chronic herbal therapy. If surgery is planned, tell your physician's that you are taking St. Johns Wort as it may interact with anesthetic agents.

Quick tip

Although popular for many years, Kava has many potentially serious side effects and should **not** be taken.

Vaginal Yeast Infections

- **Probiotics**: This treatment optimally should be used on a daily basis.
- **Echinacea**: Can be helpful for recurrent problems, particularly in combination with topical antifungal creams.
- **Tree tea oil**: Should only be used under a physician's supervision.
- **Boric acid suppositories**: Use as directed on the package.
- ➢ **My take**: For chronic problems take a daily probiotic (2-30 billion bacteria per day).

Stress and Mental Wellness

Everyone experiences varying degrees of stress whether in their job, at home, with relationships, with money problems, due to medical problems, or any other of multiple potential problems. This stress can directly impact our overall wellness, and methods to control the situation help diffuse the problem before it escalates. Each person should develop their preferred method and use this when necessary. A combination of relaxed breathing, muscle relaxation, and meditation is inexpensive and effective.

Exercise and Eating

- Eat 4-6 small "meals" per day and try to eat each meals at similar times each day
- Regular schedule of aerobic exercise (walk/bike/run/swim/etc) and anaerobic (weight lifting) is vital to overall well being. The weight lifting should be low weights with 12-15 repetitions
- Helpful for aerobic capacity, stress management, anxiety, depression, and strength level
- Cost: $

Relaxed Breathing

- Inexpensive method to manage stress
- Slowly inhale- hold- slowly exhale- then repeat
- Helpful for stress management, anxiety, nausea/vomiting, and high blood pressure
- Cost: $

Muscle Relaxation

- Sit in a quiet place and starting with the feet relax each muscle set for 30 seconds. Each session should last 10-15 minutes

- Helpful for stress management, anxiety, headaches, and high blood pressure
- Cost: $

Meditation

- Focus on breathing and repeating words or sounds. This suspends the normal thought process and allows mental and physical calmness
- Many different meditation techniques available
- Helps control emotions
- May be used in conjunction with Yoga or Tai chi
- New data suggests 3 minutes may be effective
- Helpful for stress management, fibromyalgia, chronic illness, anxiety, and high blood pressure
- Cost: $

Spirituality

- Believe in yourself and others. It is your search for the meaning of life.
- Not necessarily religious but may be
- May find this in religion, nature, art, music, community and is different for everyone
- Helpful in chronic illness, cancer, stress management, anxiety, and marriage problems
- Cost: $

Yoga

- Combines breathing and posture techniques with meditation
- Traditional Yoga combines this with dietary changes, meditation, behavior modification
- Helpful with stress management, anxiety, mood enhancement, back pain, osteoarthritis, high blood pressure, and asthma
- Cost: $$

Tai Chi

- Meditation in motion. Perform a series of postures or movements in a slow graceful motion. This improves aerobic capacity with better balance and flexibility
- Helpful for stress management, anxiety, mood enhancement, aerobic capacity, balance, depression, and high blood pressure
- Cost: $$

Art and Music Therapy

- Focusing on art or music for relaxation. Can influence physical and mental health
- Helpful for stress management, anxiety, mood enhancement, depression, Alzheimer's, and autism
- Cost: $$

Feldenkrais Method

- Similar to yoga as strives to increase flexibility and coordination and thereby creates body feedback awareness
- Helpful for stress management, anxiety, and depression
- Cost: $ to $$$

Alexander Technique

- Teaches body posture and body movement awareness. Theory is that these will influence physical well being
- Helpful for stress management, anxiety, and depression
- Minimal data available on effectiveness
- Cost: $

Massage

- Several types exist but all generally revolve around manipulation of the bodies soft tissues- skin, muscle, and tendons
- Most effective if done regularly
- Helpful for stress management, anxiety, sports soreness/injury, fibromyalgia, and chronic pain
- Rolfing is a deep muscle technique best used for sports related soreness/injury
- Best of the more expensive techniques
- Cost: $$$

Pilates

- Low impact fitness technique that improves pelvic stability and abdominal muscles. Excellent results with strengthening the back and improving posture. Also improves strength, flexibility, and joint mobility
- May use a Pilate machine or floor exercises
- Helpful for low back pain, weight loss, stress management, and anxiety
- Cost: $$

Guided Imagery/Visualization

- Visualize good places, food, etc which produces physiological, biochemical, and immunological changes
- Helpful in stress management, cancer care, anxiety
- Cost: $

Biofeedback

- Monitor heart rate, skin temperature, brain activity and teach the patient to control blood pressure, heart rate, and muscle tension
- Later learn to evoke positive responses by relaxing muscles
- Helpful for irritable bowel syndrome, stress management, anxiety, nausea/vomiting, headache, asthma, and high blood pressure

- $$$

Hypnosis

- May work through mind-body pathways in the nervous system
- Create a suggestion phase and then the person will follow these suggestion when regular consciousness is achieved
- Helpful in pain management, behavior change, anxiety, stress management, and tension headaches
- $$$

Reflexology

- Involves the theory that certain areas of your feet correspond to other parts of your body. Massage of the feet is used to correct other problems
- Unclear as to the true benefit
- Helpful for stress management, anxiety, PMS, and headaches
- $$

Quick tip

Find what method works for you and employ this in times of stress.

Treatment Techniques

Alternative treatment techniques can be a superb adjunct to regular medical treatment and physical therapy. In many situations there is not a comparable "western medicine" treatment option. As always in Integrative Medicine, a combination of western and eastern or alternative medicine may provide the optimum treatment for a particular medical condition.

Massage

- See stress and mental wellness section
- Cost: $$$

Acupuncture

- Chinese technique using the theory of Qi. Vital life energy runs along pathways called meridians. Small needles are inserted into specific points on the pathways in order to rebalance the energy flow
- Helpful for pain management, stress management, anxiety, fibromyalgia, nausea and vomiting, osteoarthritis, behavioral modification, low back pain, neck pain, irritable bowel syndrome, and GYN symptoms
- Cost: $$$

Quick tip

Acupuncture is a superb treatment regiment but does require several sessions to obtain the maximum effect and then may require a regular maintenance schedule to keep the positive effects. Make sure to find an acupuncture physician with appropriate training. A weekend course is NOT sufficient training. In many situations acupuncture is combined with a massage variant like cupping and may be combined with Chinese Herbal Therapy.

Spinal Manipulation

- Performed for Osteopathic physicians, Chiropractors, and Physical Therapists
- Theory that illness can be controlled by proper alignment of the bones, joints, muscles
- Done with both high energy and low energy techniques
- Helpful for low back pain, sports soreness/injury, headache, and neck pain
- Cost: $$$

Quick tip

Manipulation is also a very effective treatment technique and may also require multiple sessions for optimum results.

Healing touch/Therapeutic touch

- Gentle touching designed to redirect the energy flow in the body and open congested pathways
- Helpful for stress management, anxiety, chronic pain, depression, and migraines
- Cost: $$ to $$$

Reiki (Ray-kee)

- Japanese technique involving Rei which is the universal spirit and Ki which is the life force energy
- Various hand positions alter or slow the flow of energy
- Helpful for stress management, anxiety, depression, and chronic pain
- Cost: $$ to $$$

Magnetic Therapy

- Various theories on how this technique may work
- Static magnets (bracelets, shoe inserts, etc) have shown no benefit
- Electromagnetic magnets may help in bone fractures, depression, fibromyalgia, and arthritis
- Cost: $ to $$$

Smoking and Alcohol Cessation

Smoking Cessation

- **Why do people smoke:** Combination of nicotine chemical addiction with the inherent need to have something in your hands and mouth. Both facts are equally important.
- **Deleterious effects of smoking:** Increased risks of cardiac disease, strokes, peripheral vascular disease, lung disease, and multiple cancers. It is estimated that each cigarette costs 5-20 minutes of life. The great news is that stopping smoking can reverse the risks or as a minimal arrests the damage where it is.
- **Decision to stop smoking:** Only you can make the decision to stop and you must be firm in your conviction. Set a date to stop and stick to this date. Tell your family and friends and enlist their support. It is imperative that your significant other stops smoking also as it is less likely that one spouse will stop while the other continues to smoke. Make a decision whether this will be "cold turkey" or will be weaning off of cigarettes (progressively using cigarettes with lower and lower nicotine content). Decide if you will need a group for support or will if this be self help. My recommendation is cold turkey and self help with family and friend support. Finally decide if you want to use additional aids such as over the counter medications or prescription medications.
- **Tips to stop smoking:**
  1. Control your stress level. Choose a stopping date that does not include an abnormal amount of work or life stress. Set up alternatives to distract you from your desire to smoke such as additional activities, other home or work projects, meditation, etc.
  2. Will power: Plan on one day at a time. Each morning make a mental decision that you will not smoke today. 24 hours is mentally controllable whereas "never smoking again" is more difficult to accept. You must always remind yourself that you are no longer a smoker.
  3. Enlist family and friends to help. They need to know you are quitting so they offer continual support.

4. Avoid alcohol and bars, particularly in the early stages. Alcohol and smoking commonly go hand in hand. Do not put yourself in a situation where you will have higher than normal urges to smoke.
5. Keep your hands and mouth busy. Consider sunflower seeds or licorice sticks (actual twigs).
6. Brush you teeth after meals. The urge to smoke is the highest after eating and this will help control that urge.
7. Clove oil. A small drop on your fingertip and then touch it to the back of the tongue will help control smoking urges. May be used as needed.
8. Promise yourself a reward for success. Pick something you have always wanted or a trip to a dream place and reward yourself when you have successfully quit. You will be able to afford this with the money you save by not purchasing cigarettes.

- **Symptoms related to smoking cessation and suggestions to control these problems**
  1. Fatigue: Keep yourself busy, exercise, and take frequent naps
  2. Insomnia: Exercise and no caffeine after 6PM
  3. Cough: Drink plenty of fluids
  4. Dizziness/lightheadedness: Change positions slowly
  5. Poor concentration: Eat appropriately, exercise, plan your workload, use small amounts of caffeine in the morning
  6. Constipation: Push the fruits and fluids along with regular exercise
  7. Hunger: Careful with the weight gain. Eat nutritiously and stick to the lower calorie, healthy snacks
  8. Cravings: Distract yourself and concentrate on not giving in to the urges
- **Over the counter treatment options:** Very important to completely stop smoking before using any nicotine products
  1. Nicotine gum
  2. Nicotine lozenges
  3. Nicotine patch
- **Herbal supplement:** Numerous options on the Internet
  1. NicRx: may be the best option
  2. NicoCure: second best option
  3. CigArrest: starting to have questionable results
  4. CigArrette: minimal help
- **Medical treatment**

1. Hypnosis: excellent overall results. Make sure you choose a well trained hypnotist
2. Acupuncture: also excellent results and once again choose a well trained acupuncture physician

- **Pharmaceutical treatment**
  1. Zyban: Originally Wellbutrin was developed for depression treatment but this medication works extremely well for smoking cessation treatment. Used short term for 7-12 weeks.
  2. Chantix: Newest treatment available and is also used short term. Decreases the pleasurable feeling of smoking and also decreases the side effects. Currently the most popular pharmaceutical treatment.

Quick tip

Remember: Choose a date, enlist the help of friends and family, control stress levels, and have will power. These are the keys to success.

Alcohol cessation

- **Why do people drink:** Chemical addiction to alcohol, the need to party with friends and associates (although not all drunks are "fun"), the need to forget problems and stresses in their life, and the need to feel "part of the group" all play a role in why people will chronically drink alcohol.
- **Deleterious effects of alcohol:** The main, well known problem with alcohol centers on the major liver damage which can occur. In the United States, alcoholic liver disease is the number one cause of end stage liver disease and this process is insidious in nature. It is unclear as to how much alcohol intake results in advanced liver disease as each person is physiologically

different, but it is very clear that the more you drink for the greater number of years the greater the chance of liver disease. Additional damages from alcohol which are less publicized include chronic pancreatitis, CNS damage, and chronic heart disease. All of these problems can be equally devastating to your body. The great news is that the liver is able to regenerate itself to a significant degree as long as the damage is not excessive. Another reason to stop early. Remember that alcohol is alcohol and the effects are the same whether it is hard liquor, beer, or wine. 1 ½ oz of hard liquor = 5 oz of wine = 12 oz of beer = 12 oz of a wine cooler.

- **Reasons to stop drinking:**
    1. Decrease the potential health problems.
    2. Decrease the family and relationship problems.
    3. Increase productivity at work and home.
    4. Decrease legal problems. The court system does not take drunk driving offenses lightly and vehicular homicide is a major charge.
    5. Prevent harm to the baby (fetus) if you are pregnant.
    6. Save money. Alcohol is expensive.

- **Decision to stop drinking:** The first and most important facet in stopping alcohol is admitting that you are a problem drinker. Only the person with the problem can effectively realize this. Once you have come to the conclusion that alcohol is a problem then set a date to stop drinking. Make sure the chosen date does not conflict with holidays or times of increased stress as you do not want additional excuses to break your stop date. Make a decision as to what help you will require. Alcohol is a potentially dangerous drug and the physical addiction is strong. Cold turkey is generally not the answer particularly if your alcohol intake is significant. You may require medical monitoring and treatment, or as a minimum the stop date should be the date where you start to decrease your daily intake and plan on completely stopping over the course of 1-2 weeks. Consult your primary care physician before your stop date for their advice on how much medical assistance you will require.

- **Tips to stop alcohol intake:**
    1. Admit you have a problem.
    2. Set a date- consult your physician on the need for medical help.
    3. Will power: Plan on one day at a time the same as smoking cessation. Get up each morning and decide you are not going to drink today. Remind yourself you are no longer a drinker.

4. Important that your life partner does not continue to drink alcohol. It is hard to stop with other close associates continuing to drink.
5. Enlist help from family and friends. Be sure they are aware of your intentions so they will be emotionally supportive. Have your family watch closely for signs of significant alcohol withdrawal. They may notice this before you do. Make sure they are aware to inform your primary care physician immediately.
6. Avoid bars and parties where alcohol is the center piece of the event.
7. Change your social activities to decrease the peer pressure to drink. This is particularly important early on the process.
8. Consider changing the "friends" that continue to push you to drink
9. Reward yourself. Plan on purchasing something you have always wanted or go on a dream vacation once you have successfully stopped alcohol. You will be able to afford this with the money you save by not buying alcohol.

- **Physical effects of alcohol withdrawal:** May start as early as 5-10 hours or may take up to 7-10 days. Even a rapid significant decrease in alcohol intake can result in alcohol withdrawal symptoms. This is where professional medical help is needed as the side effects of withdrawal can be life threatening.
    1. Mild: Tremulousness, anxiety, irritability, fatigue, rapid emotional changes, bad dreams
    2. Moderate: Headaches, sweats, loss of appetite, increased heart rate, insomnia
    3. Severe: Seizures, DT's (delirium tremens), hallucinations, black outs
- **Help options:**
    1. Self help groups.
    2. Treatment hotlines.
    3. AA (Alcoholics Anonymous): Major advantage is having a "buddy" who has been there and understands the stresses. This person can be called when you are experiencing the urge to drink.
    4. Outpatient rehab centers.
    5. Inpatient rehab centers: May be admitted for up to 30 days.
    6. Physician's assistance: Important with almost any form of treatment. More difficult cases will require admission to an acute care hospital to complete the detoxification and control the significant alcohol withdrawal problems.

- **Nutrition:**
  1. Balanced diet: It is extremely important to plan on a well balanced diet with multiple small meals each day.
  2. Multiple vitamin with minerals. Start at least one week before alcohol cessation and continue indefinitely.
  3. Thiamine. Take 100mg per day for 3 days before you stop alcohol.
  4. Folic acid. Start one week before alcohol cessation and take 0.8mg per day for 2 months.
- **Pharmaceutical treatments:**
  1. Antabuse: Classic medication which causes severe nausea, vomiting, and abdominal pain if you attempt to drink alcohol.
  2. Zyban: The medication has been reported to curb the desire for alcohol intake.
  3. Campral
  4. Naltrexone
- **Evaluate your progress:** If you are constantly relapsing then another form of help should be considered.

Quick tip

Remember alcohol withdrawal can be potentially life threatening. Consult your primary care physician for their assistance and medical recommendations before discontinuing alcohol intake.

www.ingramcontent.com/pod-product-compliance
Lightning Source LLC
Chambersburg PA
CBHW080606270326
41928CB00016B/2942